Quality Improvement in Primary Care
The essential guide

STEPHEN GILLAM

General Practitioner, Lea Vale Medical Group, Luton
Director of Public Health Teaching, School of Clinical Medicine,
University of Cambridge

and

A NIROSHAN SIRIWARDENA

General Practitioner
Professor of Primary and Prehospital Health Care
University of Lincoln

Forewords by

PROFESSOR MARTIN ROLAND

RAND Professor of Health Services Research
Cambridge Institute of Public Health
School of Clinical Medicine, University of Cambridge

and

DR JENNIFER DIXON CE

Chief Executive
The Health Foundation

D1340100

Radcliffe Publishing
London • New York

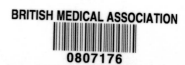

Radcliffe Publishing Ltd
St Mark's House
Shepherdess Walk
London N1 7BQ
United Kingdom

www.radcliffehealth.com

British Library Cataloguing in Publication Data

A catalogue record for this book is available from the British Library.

ISBN-13: 978 184619 768 0

The paper used for the text pages of this book
is FSC® certified. FSC (The Forest Stewardship
Council®) is an international network to promote
responsible management of the world's forests.

Typeset by Beautiful Words, Auckland, New Zealand
Manufacturing managed by 21six

Contents

Foreword by Professor Martin Roland

Quality comes and goes. When I submitted my first paper on quality to the *BMJ* in the early 1990s, the editor (in one of many rejection letters) explained that 'Our readers aren't interested in quality'. Academics have known for years that quality was important, with clear evidence in all specialties and across all countries where it has been studied that the care we give to patients often falls short of the best that could be given. Then when 25% of general practitioners' income was tied to quality through the Quality and Outcomes Framework in 2004, everyone was suddenly interested in quality (well, general practitioners at least). However, the novelty wore off and when box-ticking became overburdensome they welcomed a reduction by a third the importance of the Quality and Outcomes Framework in 2014.

Yet the simple fact remains: the care we give to patients often falls short of the best that we could give. That is despite almost all doctors and nurses going to work each day intending to do a good job. Sometimes the system conspires against them, sometimes the safeguards to prevent human error don't seem to work, and sometimes they are so worn down that 'satisfactory' seems okay and 'excellent' seems a bridge too far.

Quality improvement gurus don't always help. To be told that the error rate in manufacturing industries can be got down to one in a million is hardly motivating when you can see things going wrong all around. This excellent primer offers useful, simple practical advice: where to start, how to know how you're doing, and how to take simple steps to improve care for patients. It will be useful and used by clinicians across the health service.

Professor Martin Roland
RAND Professor of Health Services Research
Cambridge Institute of Public Health
School of Clinical Medicine, University of Cambridge
July 2014

Foreword by Dr Jennifer Dixon CBE

Training as a clinician, you would be forgiven for thinking that all there was to learn about was how best to treat patients, and perhaps their families.

However, it becomes obvious within a few months of practice that maximising the therapeutic effectiveness of your interaction with individual patients and their families may not be all that is needed to maximise the quality of care, or indeed health, for each patient. You operate within a health system, which has layers: the team, the organisation, the wider health economy, the wider health system. Just as the patient is not an island but is situated within a social, geographical, ethnic, historical or other context.

Improving the quality of care means extending the clinical purview to these wider issues, which in turn requires different skills, attitudes and approach to those learned in professional training. For example, how to influence colleagues and a wider team? How to organise care more efficiently? How best to design service improvement? How to measure impact of change? How to spread effective change? How to motivate patients to do the right thing?

Many of these issues are often classified as 'quality improvement' and often described as a science as well as an art. Quality improvement can be defined in many ways, and includes a variety of disciplines. However, at its root is the 'scientific application to everyday endeavour' – in particular, being more systematic about designing improvements needed and how they are meant to work, making small changes, testing and measuring them, and adapting change in the light of results.

The emphasis is also on continual change and improvement. For example, healthcare is not a static 'pond' – where one can test the ingredients, add more or less of something needed, and measure the result to see whether the ingredient mix is optimal – but a running river constantly in flux. Hence the emphasis is on making small changes and adapting over time as the context changes. In turn, this requires a more sophisticated, different approach to understanding the impact of service changes than traditional evaluations.

The pioneers of quality improvement – Deming, Shewhart and Juran – in fact came from other industries seeking to improve systems, reduce unwanted variation and increase the prediction of events. There is now some history in healthcare of applying the techniques they pioneered and evaluating the impact. Don Berwick and colleagues at the Institute for Healthcare Improvement in Boston have been at the forefront of these activities for at least the last quarter century, their rationale outlined in a seminal book *Curing Health Care* (Berwick, *et al.* 2002).

Since then, much of the work to date in designing, testing and evaluating impact has focused on safety and hospital care. This book fills an important gap in considering quality in primary care.

Quality Improvement in Primary Care covers the essentials, from different perspectives on quality to the practical tools for improvement and evaluating impact. It is very timely given on the one hand the increasing emphasis to reduce the need for hospitalisation through better upstream care, rising pressure from demand on primary care, and constrained resources, and on the other hand the increasing opportunities available to staff to shape general practice through commissioning or, indeed, federating practices into larger entities.

A wider challenge for the health system in the United Kingdom is how to support those in primary care wanting to trial and develop the quality improvement techniques described in this book. Opportunities are available from several organisations, including my own The Health Foundation, through grants, fellowships and leadership opportunities. The challenge will be to do this in a coordinated way and at strength over the next few years as the National Health Service in the United Kingdom faces the biggest challenges in its history.

Dr Jennifer Dixon CBE
Chief Executive
The Health Foundation
July 2014

REFERENCE

Berwick DM, Godfrey AB, Roessner J (2002) *Curing Health Care: new strategies for quality improvement; a report on the National Demonstration Project on Quality Improvement in Health Care.* Jossey-Bass: San Francisco, CA.

About the authors

Stephen Gillam
General Practitioner, Lea Vale Medical Group, Luton
Director of Public Health Teaching, School of Clinical Medicine, University of Cambridge

Stephen Gillam is a GP at the Lea Vale Medical Group in Luton and Director of Undergraduate Public Health Teaching at the University of Cambridge School of Clinical Medicine. Previously, he was Director of Primary Care at The King's Fund, where he was heavily involved in charting the impact of health policy under New Labour and developing medical managers. He is an honorary consultant at the Cambridgeshire Primary Care Trust and a visiting professor at the University of Bedfordshire.

A Niroshan Siriwardena
Professor of Primary and Prehospital Health Care, University of Lincoln, General Practitioner and Editor, Quality in Primary Care

A Niroshan Siriwardena is Professor of Primary and Prehospital Health Care at the University of Lincoln. He is a GP in Lincoln with research and teaching interests centred on quality improvement, implementation and safety science in primary and prehospital (ambulance service) care. He is editor of the journal *Quality in Primary Care*.

Introduction

Quality improvement (QI) in healthcare begins with our own personal experiences as practitioners. Every day, we encounter good care contrasted with poor or sometimes downright dangerous care. In these situations it is easy to understand why quality matters.

This primer for QI is principally directed at doctors and nurses in general practice but is relevant to all health professionals. Continuous professional development is a life-long commitment and the need for early acquisition of knowledge and skills in what is nowadays called 'quality improvement science' is compelling.

THE HISTORICAL CONTEXT FOR QUALITY IMPROVEMENT

At every stage in its development, the practice of QI has been heavily influenced by industries and activities outside the health sector. Early writers on the processes of industrial production included Ford[1] and Fayol[2] but our story really starts with Deming (Deming 1982) and Juran (Juran, *et al*. 1974). Their insights underpinned the development of total quality management. Over the past 50 years Toyota's 'lean manufacturing' and Motorola's Six Sigma have found their place in healthcare.[3]

Current approaches to risk management and patient safety – for example, in the article 'An Organisation with a Memory' (Donaldson 2002) – have borrowed heavily from the aviation industry. The idea of 'clinical governance' was derived from the private sector's concept of corporate governance (Donaldson

---

1 Frederick Winslow Taylor (1856–1915) was an early exponent of applying scientific methods to management rather than the rule-of-thumb approaches then current. He brought the skills of observation, quantification, analysis, experimentation, and evaluation to management in place of the more traditional precedent, intuition, personal opinion and guesswork.
2 The process approach to management owes much to the work of Henri Fayol (1841–1925). He focused attention on the things that a manager does, and wrote that to manage is 'to forecast and plan, to organise, to command, to coordinate and to control'. His analyses still form the basis of this 'classical view' of management.
3 The lean technique entails assessing every process for its value to the patient, to cut waste and inefficiencies and improve patient care. Six Sigma describes the aspiration to reduce error rates to the extremely low level of 3.4 per million. The term Six Sigma comes from a statistical measure of variation, the standard deviation from a normal distribution. The number of 3.4 million comes from the limits for acceptable quality being set to include all observations within six standard deviations of the mean. The statistical terminology can be confusing, but the idea is simple: we should not accept the current common error rates of 50% in healthcare, nor 10% or even 1%, but strive for near-perfect error rates of less than 1 in 3.4 million. Proponents of Six Sigma argue that these error rates are achievable in healthcare, just as in manufacturing, and cite anaesthesia as an example of an area that has seen dramatic improvements in safety.

1998). The current emphasis on health systems – 'every system is designed to achieve the results it gets' – is an important development because it moves improvement from individuals to organisations and their leaders (Nolan 1998).

Organisations such as the Institute for Healthcare Improvement in the United States, and previously the National Health Service (NHS) Institute for Innovation and Improvement in the United Kingdom, have championed improvement science and these novel approaches in healthcare (Berwick 1998).

THE SOCIAL CONTEXT

Demographic change is a major driver of increasing demand for healthcare. By 2020, one in four of the population will be aged 65 years and older, rising from one in six today. On average, people in this age group consume five times the national average of health resources. At an individual level, care at the end of life constitutes about three-quarters of all healthcare consumed over a lifespan (National Audit Office 2008).

Chronic conditions are the major causes of disability and death, and people affected by these consume the majority of healthcare resources in developed countries. Most healthcare systems are still designed to deal primarily with acute health problems and lack an effective chronic care model.

At the same time, people want more choice and greater control of health services. The future is likely to see more involvement of people in the public services they use – greater weight accorded to their views and the end of deference to health professionals and bureaucracy.

THE POLITICAL CONTEXT

Sadly, much of the political momentum for change over the last 20 years has derived from well-publicised scandals: Bristol, Alder Hey, Shipman, Mid Staffordshire – these names are engraved on the collective consciousness of the public and professionals alike. Each in turn was followed by major inquiries. The Kennedy report examined the events surrounding the death of over 30 babies after paediatric heart surgery at the Bristol Royal Infirmary. Its recommendations (*see* Box 0.1) drove major changes in the way medical practice is overseen (Kennedy 2001).

With the publication of its White Paper, *A First Class Service*, the New Labour government of the time placed QI at the centre of the health policy stage (Department of Health 1998). The term 'clinical governance' was used to capture the range of activities required to improve the quality of health services together with accountability for their delivery. Central among these were the need for all NHS organisations to develop processes for continuously monitoring and improving quality and to develop systems of accountability to ensure these were in place.

Components of clinical governance include evidence-based practice, clinical audit, risk management, mechanisms to monitor the outcomes of care, lifelong learning, and systems for managing poor performance. In addition, the term combines an emphasis on improving care for individual patients with QI targeted at whole populations.

BOX 0.1 Bristol Royal Infirmary inquiry – key concerns

- The need for clearly understood clinical standards
- How clinical competence and technical expertise are assessed and evaluated
- The reliability and validity of data used to monitor doctors' personal performance
- The appreciation of the importance of non-clinical factors affecting clinical performance
- The responsibility of a consultant to take appropriate actions in responses to concerns about his or her performance
- The factors that seem to discourage openness and frankness about doctors' personal performance
- How doctors explain risks to patients
- The ways in which people concerned about patients' safety can make their concerns known
- The need for doctors to take prompt action at an early stage when a colleague is in difficulty, to avoid damage to patients

---

THE SCIENTIFIC CONTEXT

Medical scientific knowledge and the evidence for what works, its costs and safety are increasing at an exponential rate. Practitioners have to rely on the translation of evidence to systematic reviews and guidance rather than necessarily having time to access primary sources of research. Archie Cochrane, who first extolled the importance of the randomised controlled trial, is often regarded as the father of evidence-based healthcare. Successors such as David Sackett and Iain Chalmers established his lasting legacy in the Cochrane Centre, which coordinates the production and publication of high-quality systematic reviews.

Our ability to deliver safe, effective healthcare is struggling to keep up with the rapid advances in science and medical treatments. Constraints on how best to exploit the revolution in information technology is just one of the reasons why (Institute of Medicine 2001).

The translation of guidance into routine practice is one of the greatest challenges for healthcare – the so-called 'second translation gap'. QI provides a means to bridge this gap and so the science of QI is now as essential to good practice as the anatomy, biochemistry and physiology that doctors and other health workers learn in their undergraduate training.

WHAT DO WE MEAN BY QUALITY?

There are three key models of quality in current use. Avedis Donabedian, in his classic paper 'Evaluating the Quality of Medical Care', first enunciated the quality triad of structure, process and outcome (Donabedian 1966). This formed the basic structure for medical audit activity in the 1980s, symbolically redefined as 'clinical audit' in acknowledgement of the multidisciplinary nature of all QI activities.

The Institute of Medicine's *Crossing the Quality Chasm: A New Health System for the 21st Century* was a landmark report on quality from the United States, identifying effectiveness, efficiency, safety, timeliness and patient-centredness as key dimensions of quality (Institute of Medicine 2001). In the United States these have been refined into the 'triple aim' of improving the experience of care, improving the health of populations, and reducing per capita costs of health-care (Berwick, *et al.* 2008). In the United Kingdom the *Next Stage Review* refined these to safety, effectiveness (and efficiency) and patient experience (Darzi of Denham 2008).

A number of other conceptual frameworks provide further ways of thinking about quality in primary care. Toon's (1994) exploration of 'good general prac-tice' distinguished three different approaches: (1) a disease-focused, biomedical model; (2) a patient-focused, humanist model; and (3) a population-focused, public health model. Toon argued that the meaning of good general practice differs between these three models and that this helps to explain the variety of approaches to assessing and improving quality that have been put forward.

Howie, *et al.* (1997) attempted to assess quality from the patient's perspec-tive by measuring the extent to which the consultation enables the patient to understand and cope with his or her illness. McColl, *et al.* (1998) took a more biomedical approach, proposing that primary care teams can assess the potential impact of different clinical activities by applying evidence on clini-cal effectiveness as performance indicators to their own practice population. Roland, *et al.* (1998) combined patient, population and organisational per-spectives to identify 14 markers of quality in general practice. These included measures of access and availability (e.g. waiting times and telephone access to doctors); clinical markers relating to the quality of acute, chronic, terminal and preventive care; and measures of prescribing and referrals. They provided the basis upon which the Quality and Outcomes Framework was constructed (*see* Chapter 9) (Gillam and Siriwardena 2010).

Greenhalgh and Eversely (1999) explored five different perspectives from which to consider quality in general practice. They distinguished patient, activ-ity and performance, evidence-based, educational and managerial perspectives, each of which focuses on a different cluster of markers of quality. They argued that no single perspective can be used to describe quality of care. In a simi-lar vein, Toon (1994) argued that it is impossible to define a single version of good-quality general practice if there is no agreement on what it is aiming to achieve and the values it is promoting. These points are relevant to clinical commissioning groups in the United Kingdom, whose key tasks are develop-ing primary care services, commissioning healthcare and improving the health of the local population (*see* Chapter 4). This combination of individual and population-based goals needs to be reflected in the range of clinical governance activities that underpins them.

WHAT DRIVES QUALITY IMPROVEMENT?

The main drivers of QI and healthcare are threefold and interrelated.

1 **Education.** At one time doctors and nurses were thought to emerge 'fully formed' from medical and nursing schools. In our professional lifetimes, it was possible to go straight from pre-registration house jobs to take on all the responsibilities of general practice without any higher training. As train-ing programmes have evolved in terms of their breadth and sophistication, the notion of time-bounded clinical education has faded. Clinical (includ-ing medical) education is a career-long, continuous process, central to the

maintenance and improvement of quality. In the third section of this book, we will examine how you need to approach this challenge.

2 **Health service evaluation and audit.** All health professionals need to understand how to measure quality; they are all directly or indirectly involved in evaluating the quality of the services they provide. The motives for doing so are not simply altruistic. In our litigious age, practitioners need not only to understand how to deal with complaints but also to pre-empt medico-legal consequences of health service failures. The main driver, however, is surely internal and linked to an ethos of professionalism. For most doctors, job satisfaction is largely derived from delivering services they perceive to be optimal. We wish to do as we would be done by.

3 **Market mechanisms, choice and regulation.** The third set of drivers to improve quality relate to market (financial) incentives, choice and regulation. There is a long history of using payment to improve the quality of general practice in the United Kingdom (UK). Evidence for their effectiveness is contested, but the elements of successful pay-for-performance schemes can be delineated (*see* Chapter 9). A closely related consideration is patient choice. In an unfettered market, consumer choice of healthcare provider is supposed to be based in large measure on perceptions of quality. Central to this is the provision of meaningful information to users about quality of care and, of course, the ability to make real choices (*see* Chapter 1). These are not 'givens' in a state-run monolith such as the NHS, and successive government reforms have sought to strengthen consumer power, through greater involvement and choice, and also to ensure that regulation helps to safeguard the consumer. The recent restructuring of the health service and legislative changes will see regulatory organisations such as the Care Quality Commission and Monitor assuming increased powers in the coming years (*see* Chapter 3).

WHOSE BUSINESS IS IT ANYWAY?

Health service commissioners, currently clinical commissioning groups in England, are the organisations through which clinical governance will be developed at a local level and local priorities identified. However, the members of individual practices and primary care teams undertake the nitty-gritty work of clinical governance and QI.

Over the last two decades consideration of the 'primary care team' has begun to replace narrower discussions about general practice, but there is no single definition of the scope or constituency of primary care. In the UK, the term is often used interchangeably with general practice. Therefore, most work on quality focuses on general practice.

Underpinning contemporary theories of QI is the axiom that poor individual performance usually reflects wider 'system failure' or the absence of an organisation-wide system of quality assurance. In healthcare organisations, critical incidents can lead to death, disability or permanent discomfort. This, together with the tendency of clinicians to protect their individual autonomy and reputation, can promote a culture of blame and secrecy that inhibits the organisational learning necessary to prevent such incidents in the future.

Introducing clinical governance to primary care, the government stated that it must be seen as a systematic approach to quality assurance and improvement within a health organisation . . . Above all clinical governance is about changing organisational culture . . . away from a culture of blame to one of learning so that quality infuses all aspects of the organisation's work. (Donaldson and Gray 1998)

Therefore, organisational development is central to the effective establishment of clinical governance.

STRUCTURE OF THIS BOOK

We begin Section 1 of *Quality Improvement in Primary Care* by considering how to manage primary care organisations in order to improve quality of care. We start, as we always should, with our patients' perspectives on quality and how to measure these.

As we have seen, the concept of clinical governance places a central responsibility for quality on the shoulders of those managing and leading within the health system. To one degree or another, that means all of us. Leadership, management and the right organisational culture are prerequisites for improvement. How these can support QI is examined next. All doctors and other healthcare practitioners work within teams, organisations and the wider health system; how these are designed and managed greatly determines both an individual's and a team's effectiveness.

We go on to examine market mechanisms and commissioning, which are increasingly being used as levers for change. We conclude this section by considering how general practices are regulated and held accountable for the quality of the services they provide.

In Section 2 we look in more detail at the techniques used for assessing and measuring quality of care. In many ways, this constitutes the practical core of the book. It is one thing to observe (or diagnose) and another thing to effect change (or cure). We explore how QIs are actually delivered. The tools described in each of these chapters are illustrated with case examples. We look at commonly used frameworks for QI – for example, the clinical audit cycle, the plan-do-study-act cycle and significant event analysis – before considering how quality is measured. We introduce the burgeoning sciences of process control, systems and spread. This section concludes with a chapter on the evaluation of quality.

In Section 3 we return to our own needs as individual practitioners. Nowadays, preparing for and acting on appraisal is a regular feature of clinicians' working lives. How do we provide care that reflects the most up-to-date evidence? How do we identify our own developmental needs and work with others to address them? This is not just about providing more satisfactory experiences for the people we serve. It is also about deepening the personal yields from what is already a rewarding occupation. Throughout the text we suggest prompts for reflection and each chapter includes case studies. What do you, the reader, want to provide and receive from your work?

CONCLUSION

Our aim in *Quality Improvement in Primary Care* is to provide readers with a set of tools to convert the endless challenges for quality and myriad opportunities for improvement into meaningful and useful change. We hope to enable you as practitioners to use your personal experiences to transform the services you provide. It is not possible to cover all aspects of this topic – we do not cover detailed statistics, for example – but we have pointed readers to other relevant resources. We hope, nevertheless, that this book provides an introductory primer for QI, relevant to every individual working and learning in primary healthcare and the wider health service who needs to understand what QI is and how QI should be carried out . . . that means *all of us*.

REFERENCES

Berwick DM (1998) Developing and testing changes in delivery of care. *Ann Intern Med.* **128**(8): 651–6.

Berwick DM, Nolan TW, Whittington J (2008) The triple aim: care, health, and cost. *Health Aff (Millwood).* **27**(3): 759–69.

Darzi of Denham AD (2008) *High quality care for all: NHS Next Stage Review final report.* CM 7432. The Stationery Office: London.

Deming WE (1982) *Out of the crisis.* Massachusetts Institute of Technology, Center for Advanced Engineering Study: Cambridge, MA.

Department of Health (1998) *A first class service: quality in the new NHS.* Department of Health: London.

Donabedian A (1966) Evaluating the quality of medical care. *Milbank Mem Fund Q.* **44**(3 Suppl.): 166–206.

Donaldson L (2002) An organisation with a memory. *Clin Med.* **2**(5): 452–7.

Donaldson LJ (1998) Clinical governance: a statutory duty for quality improvement. *J Epidemiol Community Health.* **52**(2): 73–4.

Donaldson LJ, Gray JA (1998) Clinical governance: a quality duty for health organisations. *Qual Health Care.* **7**(Suppl.): S37–44.

Gillam S, Siriwardena AN (2010) *The Quality and Outcomes Framework: QOF transforming general practice.* Radcliffe Publishing: Oxford.

Greenhalgh T, Eversley J (1999) *Quality in general practice: towards a holistic approach.* The King's Fund: London.

Howie JG, Heaney DJ, Maxwell M (1997) Measuring quality in general practice: pilot study of a needs, process and outcome measure. *Occas Pap R Coll Gen Pract.* (75): i–xii, 1–32.

Institute of Medicine (2001) *Crossing the quality chasm: a new health system for the 21st century.* The National Academies Press: Washington, DC.

Juran JM, Gryna FM, Bingham RS (1974) *Quality control handbook.* McGraw-Hill: New York, NY.

Kennedy I (2001) *Learning from Bristol: the report of the public inquiry into children's heart surgery at the Bristol Royal Infirmary 1984–1995.* The Stationery Office: London.

McColl A, Roderick P, Gabbay J, et al. (1998) Performance indicators for primary care groups: an evidence based approach. *BMJ.* **317**(7169): 1354–60.

National Audit Office (2008) *End of life care.* The Stationery Office: London.

Nolan TW (1998) Understanding medical systems. *Ann Intern Med.* **128**(4): 293–8.

Roland M, Holden J, Campbell S (1998) *Quality assessment for general practice: supporting clinical governance in primary care groups.* National Primary Care Research and Development Centre: Manchester.

Toon PD (1994) *What is good general practice?* Royal College of General Practitioners: London.

Managing for quality

CHAPTER 1

Patient perspectives

SUMMARY

- Perspectives of service users, patients and carers, and the public are central to quality improvement in healthcare.
- Service users are increasingly involved in generating information to guide others seeking healthcare, helping to determine needs or preferences in healthcare choices, and providing feedback on health services.
- Measures of patient satisfaction, patient experience and patient-reported outcomes are closely related but different ways of expressing the quality of health services from a patient perspective.
- The different methods of collecting patient and carer feedback – including surveys, measures or interviews – have advantages and disadvantages.
- Patients and the public will in future have greater involvement in commissioning, monitoring and regulation, with an increasing role in improving and redesigning health services.

THE PATIENT PERSPECTIVE

In this first chapter we focus on patient perspectives on healthcare quality improvement and how we might involve patients, carers and the public in developing our notions of quality, in supporting quality improvement efforts, and in monitoring and regulating services. Throughout this book we will emphasise the primary importance of patients' perspectives on quality. Indeed, it could be reasonably asked, what perspective of quality is there other than the patient viewpoint, whether this relates to the care that the patient experiences or the clinical outcomes that result?

Joseph Juran defined quality in two ways: first, 'those features of products which meet customer needs and thereby provide customer satisfaction'; second, 'freedom from deficiencies' (Juran and Godfrey 1999). However, Deming (1982) makes the point that quality depends on who is the judge of quality. In the case of healthcare this could be the patient, healthcare professional, manager, organisation, commissioner, inspector or regulator, each with his, her or its own perspective. As information about healthcare interventions, professionals and organisations improve, as it becomes more available and presented more clearly, and as public involvement at various levels increases, service users will play a greater role as judges of quality.

Understanding what service users value is therefore necessary, but not always sufficient, for knowing where we should focus quality improvement efforts. Just as importantly, service users should be involved in how we should bring improvement about or judge whether it has been achieved. This requires a major shift in our thinking from patients being (passive) recipients of care to being (actively) involved in informing and improving services.

Unfortunately, in the past, quality and improvement efforts in healthcare have focused on what professionals think patients should value, and have been less interested in what service users themselves feel is important or have failed to elicit patients' views directly. Professional perspectives are a proxy for that of the patient but there may be occasions where the two diverge and the reasons for this need to be understood.

Recent major failures in health services – for example, those described in the Francis report, detailing widely publicised failures at a hospital in Stafford in central England – have reiterated the importance of the patient perspective (Francis 2010).

To quote Robert Francis QC:

> [It is the] individual experiences that lie behind statistics and benchmarks and action plans that really matter, and that is what must never be forgotten when policies are being made and implemented. (Francis 2010)

Clinicians, managers or commissioners of services may all try to see issues from the patient perspective and claim to represent patients. However, the focus of this chapter is the involvement of service users themselves and their representatives in measuring satisfaction, experience or outcomes, in making judgements about the quality of services, and in designing improvements in healthcare.

Points to ponder
- How do you currently gather information on patient preferences, satisfaction, experiences and outcomes for your service?
- How would you describe the most recent judgements from service users on your service, and what was your response?

QUALITY FRAMEWORKS AND PATIENT VIEWS OF SERVICES

Many well-known quality frameworks highlight the importance of patient experience. For example, the US Institute of Medicine, in their landmark monograph *Crossing the Quality Chasm: A New Health System for the 21st Century*, referred to patient-centredness together with safety, timeliness, effectiveness, efficiency and equity as the fundamental components of quality (Institute of Medicine 2001). 'Patient-centredness' is a complex term that means different things to different people (Siriwardena and Norfolk 2007), but in this context it refers to respect for an individual patient's culture, social context and specific needs and it encourages the patient to be active in decisions about his or her own care.

In the UK, efforts are being made to identify and address the key quality issues for health systems in terms of the triad of safety, effectiveness and experience (Darzi of Denham 2008). This has led to a renewed focus on improving patient outcomes (Department of Health 2010). The National Health Service (NHS) Outcomes Framework has 'ensuring people have a positive experience of care' as one of five outcome domains (Department of Health 2013b). The NHS Constitution lays down the rights (and responsibilities) of its patients and staff in order to achieve this (Department of Health 2013a). Recent studies have suggested that there is a consistent positive relationship between patient experience, effectiveness and safety (Doyle, *et al.* 2013), reinforcing the importance of patient experience as part of the quality triad.

More recently, in response to the review of failures at the Mid Staffordshire NHS Foundation Trust, Don Berwick and the National Advisory Group on the Safety of Patients in England, in their publication *A Promise to Learn – a Commitment to Act: Improving the Safety of Patients in England*, expressed that patients and carers should be present, powerful, and involved at all levels of healthcare organisations (National Advisory Group on the Safety of Patients in England 2013). Finally, the Keogh review, or *Review into the Quality of Care and Treatment Provided by 14 Hospital Trusts in England*, stated that we should involve patients, carers and members of the public as vital and equal partners in design of services and involve patients and clinicians as active participants in regulatory inspections (Keogh 2013).

Points to ponder
- What have been the recent failures in the service you provide or in provision of services you were aware of?
- What were these failures due to and how might they have been prevented?
- What might the role of service users have been in preventing failures and how could service user input be better used in future?

PATIENT PREFERENCES, SATISFACTION, EXPERIENCE AND OUTCOMES

Patient preferences, satisfaction, experience and outcomes (*see* Table 1.1) are overlapping but not identical concepts. Satisfaction and experience are both expressions of 'utility' or 'happiness' with services provided. Of course, many people prefer not to use services unless they have to.

There are many ways of eliciting patient views, ranging from those such as surveys or questionnaires, which attempt to provide a broader more representative assessment from the population being sampled, to interviews, focus groups and patient stories, which try to gain a more in-depth understanding. Other methods that provide lesser degrees of breadth and depth of views include online ratings, 'mystery shoppers', complaints and compliments from patients, relatives or friends, feedback from patient liaison services or patient participation groups, and public meetings (De Silva 2013).

Patient satisfaction surveys are regularly undertaken in most health settings and are intended to provide a quantitative (and often representative) assessment of satisfaction with services in a number of domains. For example, the general practice patient survey linked to the Quality and Outcomes Framework (Gillam and Siriwardena 2010) covers areas such as access (telephone, face-to-face, in-hours, out-of-hours), continuity, communication, care (from the

TABLE 1.1 Measuring patient preferences, satisfaction, experience and outcomes

	Preferences	Satisfaction	Experience	Outcomes
Instruments	Interviews, focus groups, surveys, consensus methods (nominal group, Delphi), or experiments (e.g. discrete choice experiments)	Satisfaction survey	PREM; interviews or narrative interviews (patient stories)	Patient-reported outcome or outcome measure
Timing	Before or after	After	After	After, when compared with threshold score, or before-and-after
Advantages	Help inform decisions about provision of services	Easy to administer and analyse	PREMs easy to administer and analyse; interviews	Valid and reliable outcome measures are available for a range of conditions or generic health status (e.g. EQ-5D)
Disadvantages	Problematic when trying to elicit future needs or preferences; results can vary according to method and population	Poorly constructed questions, selective distribution and/or low response rates can lead to bias; positive overall ratings can mask significant problems of experience	Expensive to develop valid and reliable PREMs or to conduct and analyse interviews; poorly constructed questions, selective distribution and/or low response rates can lead to bias	Expensive to develop valid and reliable measures, and to administer and analyse; many conditions do not have appropriate measures developed

PREM = patient-related experience measure

general practitioner, nurse or receptionist), support for self-care and overall satisfaction (Carter, *et al.* 2009). The questions and response formats are constrained by particular areas and issues that are considered to be important for service provision and patient satisfaction.

Satisfaction levels with health services, particularly general practice, are often high, but this does not necessarily mean that users' experiences of services are good. Surveys can be biased by how they are administered: high satisfaction with access in patients distributed a survey in a general practice waiting room may hide poor levels of satisfaction in those patients having the greatest difficulty getting appointments. Questions may be focused on what health professionals think constitutes a good experience, which is not necessarily the same as what patients perceive or need. Finally, satisfaction will be affected by patients' expectations (Black and Jenkinson 2009).

For example, a focus group study showed how the complexities of patients' wants and needs from a consultation for insomnia differed from what doctors thought they wanted or needed (*see* Box 1.1) (Dyas, *et al.* 2010). This understanding has been translated into an e-learning programme for doctors, nurses and other health professionals (Siriwardena 2014).

UNDERSTANDING THE PATIENT EXPERIENCE

To understand patients' experiences implies seeking to see things from the perspective of patients. This requires us to work with patients to gather information on what constitutes a good or a poor experience, and this may vary by person and setting. In the UK, the Department of Health has tried to address what domains of experience might look like through a patient experience framework, derived from those developed by the Institute of Medicine and the

---

BOX 1.1 Case study – patient and views on improving primary care for insomnia

The authors conducted a focus group of patients with insomnia and general practitioners caring for those with sleep problems to elicit preferences for care. Patients with insomnia initially tried to resolve the problem themselves and consulting a general practitioner was often a last resort. Patients felt they needed to convince practitioners that their sleep difficulties were serious. They described insomnia in terms of the impact it was having on their life, whereas clinicians tended to focus on underlying causes.

Patients wanted to be shown understanding, to be listened to and to be taken seriously. What they initially saw as a lifestyle problem had become 'medicalised', often leading to a request for a hypnotic prescription. Doctors felt that patients might not take non-drug treatments seriously and expected patients to be resistant to stopping drugs they were already taking or reluctant to explore alternatives, whereas patients, often deriving little benefit from drugs, were open to alternatives such as psychological therapies.

Better management of insomnia should take into account the perceptions and interactions of patients and practitioners. Practitioners need to empathise, listen, elicit patients' beliefs and expectations, assess sleep better and offer a range of treatments, including cognitive and behavioural therapies, tailored to individual needs.

(Dyas, *et al.* 2010)

Picker Institute (*see* Box 1.2) (Department of Health 2011).

Over the past few years, psychologists have begun to distinguish between the memory of an experience and the experience as it happens, since what we usually refer to as experience is what we remember of the experience. This might seem an artificial distinction until we appreciate that our memory of an experience is affected not only by what happens during it but also by the peak experience (of pleasure or pain) and how the experience ends. If the peak experience is highly positive and particularly if it ends well this increases our likelihood of recollecting this to be a good experience (Kahneman 2012).

Healthcare providers, commissioners, regulators and service users are increasingly seeing patient-related experience measures and patient-reported outcome measures as important tools (Black and Jenkinson 2009). Patient-related experience measures are brief questionnaires developed to measure people's experiences of services, whereas patient-reported outcome measures are short, self-completed questionnaires that measure health status, health-related quality of life or experience of care at a point in time. Patient-reported outcome measures change over time (pre and post intervention), which allows the impact of healthcare interventions to be assessed (Black and Jenkinson 2009). Outcomes have been found to be correlated with but not distinct from experience (Sequist, *et al.* 2008). The National Institute for Health and Care Excellence in the United Kingdom has also developed statements on what constitutes good experience in adult services (*see* Box 1.3) (National Institute for Health and Clinical Excellence 2012).

BOX 1.2 National Health Service patient experience framework

- Respect for patient-centred values, preferences, and expressed needs, including cultural issues; the dignity, privacy and independence of patients and service users; an awareness of quality-of-life issues; and shared decision-making
- Coordination and integration of care across the health and social care system
- Information, communication, and education on clinical status, progress, prognosis, and processes of care in order to facilitate autonomy, self-care and health promotion
- Physical comfort including pain management, help with activities of daily living, and clean and comfortable surroundings
- Emotional support and alleviation of fear and anxiety about such issues as clinical status, prognosis and the impact of illness on patients, their families and their finances
- Welcoming the involvement of family and friends, on whom patients and service users rely, in decision-making and demonstrating awareness and accommodation of their needs as caregivers
- Transition and continuity as regards information that will help patients care for themselves away from a clinical setting, and coordination, planning and support to ease transitions
- Access to care with attention, for example, to time spent waiting for admission or time between admission and placement in a room in an inpatient setting, and waiting time for an appointment or visit in the outpatient, primary care or social care setting.

(Department of Health 2011)

BOX 1.3 National Institute for Health and Care Excellence quality statements on adult patient experience

- Patients are treated with dignity, kindness, compassion, courtesy, respect, understanding and honesty.
- Patients experience effective interactions with staff who have demonstrated competency in relevant communication skills.
- Patients are introduced to all healthcare professionals involved in their care, and are made aware of the roles and responsibilities of the members of the healthcare team.
- Patients have opportunities to discuss their health beliefs, concerns and preferences to inform their individualised care.
- Patients are supported by healthcare professionals to understand relevant treatment options, including benefits, risks and potential consequences.
- Patients are actively involved in shared decision-making and supported by healthcare professionals to make fully informed choices about investigations, treatment and care that reflect what is important to them.
- Patients are made aware that they have the right to choose, accept or decline treatment and these decisions are respected and supported.
- Patients are made aware that they can ask for a second opinion.
- Patients experience care that is tailored to their needs and personal preferences, taking into account their circumstances, their ability to access services and their coexisting conditions.
- Patients have their physical and psychological needs regularly assessed and addressed, including nutrition, hydration, pain relief, personal hygiene and anxiety.
- Patients experience continuity of care delivered, whenever possible, by the same healthcare professional or team throughout a single episode of care.
- Patients experience coordinated care with clear and accurate information exchange between relevant health and social care professionals.
- Patients' preferences for sharing information with their partner, family members and/or carers are established, respected and reviewed throughout their care.
- Patients are made aware of who to contact, how to contact them and when to make contact about their ongoing healthcare needs.

(National Institute for Health and Clinical Excellence 2012)

The different methods for accessing patient views have their pros and cons. These include issues of selection and reporting bias, representativeness, depth, complexity of analysis, and the level of expertise and analysis and amount of time required (De Silva 2013). Qualitative feedback is sometimes more valuable than exhaustive quantitative surveys, but often a combination of both are required to understand experiences in depth and to compare and improve services.

Finally, although much effort is nowadays expended in collecting data on patient experience, the evidence that this has led to much service improvement is, as yet, disappointing. A concerted attempt is needed to ensure these data are used to good effect (Coulter, *et al.* 2014).

Points to ponder
- How would you describe the difference between satisfaction and experience?
- Which methods would you use for measuring satisfaction or experience?

PATIENT INVOLVEMENT

Involving patients to access their views and to implement improvements is something that health services are at an early stage of addressing. Users can be individual patients, patient group members or patient representatives, each with different levels and kinds of knowledge, experience or approach, which might lead to conflicting views (Williamson 2007). There are demands from government and health organisations to increase patient involvement and, despite some validated tools and much accumulated experience, tools, structures, strategies and methods for involving patients are still being developed (Wiig, *et al.* 2013).

For example, *Transforming Participation in Health and Care* sets out a grand vision for participation in the UK NHS. It provides a framework for commissioners of services to promote individual participation in care, to engage the public in commissioning, to act upon patient feedback, to engage with patients, carers and the public when redesigning health services, and to publish evidence of these activities and their impact on services (NHS England 2013).

Patient participation groups (PPGs) are well established in many practices (Nagraj and Gillam 2011). Activities and roles undertaken by PPGs can be grouped into three categories: the first concerns health education (e.g. running educational meetings for patients); the second is the role of 'critical friend', giving advice and feedback on services provided by the practice; for the third, some groups generate material support for practice developments (e.g. through fundraising or providing voluntary services). In 2011, new financial incentives were introduced to promote the establishment of PPGs but they remain difficult to sustain. The two most important determinants of success are strong leadership and enthusiasm for the group's work by the members themselves. Committed support from the practice team and a willingness to listen to sometimes unpalatable 'home truths' are also necessary if PPGs are to effect change.

Regulation is another area where the public are increasingly involved. For example, there is now greater lay and patient involvement in regulatory bodies (such as the Care Quality Commission, Monitor and professional bodies in the United Kingdom), regulatory inspections and appraisal of health workers, and this is likely to increase in future.

Point to ponder
- How could you involve patients, their relatives, carers or the general public in improving the services you provide?

WHY CONTINUITY OF CARE MATTERS

General practitioners are nowadays more likely to work in larger practices, with the proportion of single-handed providers having dropped to 1809 (21.7%) in 2010 from 2662 (29.7%) in 2000 (NHS Information Centre 2011). General practice is becoming more organisationally complex in terms of the diversity of activities undertaken and staff employed, let alone the information technology support and premises required. This places a disproportionate burden on small practices. However, patient satisfaction is often higher in practices with fewer doctors, notably in relation to continuity of care. There is good evidence that patients are more satisfied when they see the same doctor (Saultz and Albedaiwi 2004).

Incidentally, an analogous trend towards economies of scale can be seen in the hospital sector, where there is increasing evidence that surgeons undertaking small volumes of specialised activity may have poorer outcomes. This has led to the concentration of tertiary activities such as paediatric cardiac surgery in fewer, highly specialised units.

Continuity of care refers to how an individual's healthcare is connected over time (Guthrie, *et al.* 2008). Continuity is of less concern to young healthy people consulting with minor, acute problems. However, for patients with chronic, more serious conditions, there is general agreement that continuity matters across all three of its core dimensions: informational, management and (in particular) relationship continuity (*see* Box 1.4) (Haggerty, *et al.* 2003). There is less agreement about which dimensions matter most, or the right balance between continuity and access, but an effective healthcare organisation needs to embody all dimensions of continuity, alongside good access and systematic care.

Patients who have chronic disease(s) particularly value relationship continuity, for reasons of efficiency (not having to repeat complex histories) and effectiveness (the relationship allows for greater involvement in decision-making). They trust that their doctor will take responsibility for their current and future care (Guthrie and Wyke 2006). Michael Balint identified the importance of responsibility in the 1950s. He described the 'collusion of anonymity', where general practitioners and specialists avoid taking responsibility for complex patients who attend both, each assuming that the patient is the other's problem (Balint 1957). In the face of increasingly fragmented care, Balint's conclusion remains true: generalists are best placed to take responsibility for holistic care, coordination and advocacy for the most complex patients. That generalist is usually a doctor, but increasingly nurses and case managers may take on this role.

Although neglected by policymakers, relationship continuity remains important, both because it matters to patients and because it is surely a source of efficiency. Detailed knowledge of your patients' past history can obviate the need for onward referral. One response has been the advanced medical home model, proposed by the American College of Physicians. This model promotes systems of access whereby patients get traditional, personal care from a known doctor with responsibility for coordinating all of their care, to ensure that it is coherent, integrated and effective (Barr and Ginsburg 2006).

BOX 1.4 Three types of continuity of care (Guthrie, *et al.* 2008)

1 Informational continuity: formally recorded information is complemented by tacit knowledge of patient preferences, values and context that is usually held in the memory of clinicians with whom the patient has an established relationship

2 Management continuity: shared management plans or care protocols, and explicit responsibility for follow-up and coordination, provide a sense of predictability and security in future care for both patients and providers

3 Relationship continuity: built on accumulated knowledge of patient preferences and circumstances that is rarely recorded in formal records and interpersonal trust based on experience of past care and positive expectations of future competence and care

---

COMMUNICATING RISK

Risks may be voluntary or imposed, they may be familiar or unknown and they may be concentrated or dispersed over time. These characteristics affect the way people interpret information on risk, and the way they discount the risks over time affects their responses to them. A whole range of so-called 'fright factors' characterise those risks we fear most (*see* Box 1.5). The common thread linking most of these factors is loss of control. For example, Creutzfeldt–Jakob disease is terrifying because it seems to strike arbitrarily, affecting young people and resulting in total loss of bodily control. It remains poorly understood, as reflected in uncertain statements from government. People's interpretations of a condition and its burden also vary – for example, fear of having a stroke will mean different things to different people, according to their personal experience.

BOX 1.5 'Fright factors' – what characterises those risks we fear most?

- Do not involve voluntary choice
- Cannot escape by taking personal precautions
- Unfamiliar or novel
- Man-made rather than natural
- Hidden and irreversible
- Danger to children and future generations
- Dreadful outcome
- Poorly understood by science
- Subject to contradictory statements
- Cause damage to identifiable victims

Risk communication is defined as the open two-way exchange of information and opinion about risk, leading to better understanding and better decisions about clinical management (Edwards, *et al.* 2000). This definition moves away from the notion that information is communicated only from clinician to patient, and that the acceptability (or not) of the risk is communicated back.

The two-way exchange about information and opinion is important if decisions about treatment are to reflect the attitudes to risk of the people who will live with the outcomes.

THE PROBLEMS OF RISK LANGUAGE

Terms such as 'probable', 'unlikely' and 'rare' have been shown to convey elastic concepts (Budescu, *et al.* 1988). One person's understanding of 'likely' may be a chance of one in ten, whereas another may think that it means a chance of one in two. Any one person may also interpret the term differently in different contexts: a 'rare' outcome is a different prospect in the context of genetic or antenatal tests than, for example, in the context of antibiotic treatment for tonsillitis.

Further problems in communicating risks result from the effects of different information frames (*see* Box 1.6). Logically equivalent choice situations can be presented in different ways, such as advising patients about their prognosis by using either survival or mortality data.

BOX 1.6 Choices depend on how risk is communicated

One hundred and forty senior managers were asked which of four cardiac rehabilitation programmes they would implement (Fahey *et al.* 1995). These are the data they were given about the relative effectiveness of the programmes. During a 3-year follow-up:
- programme A reduced the rate of death by 20%
- programme B produced an absolute reduction in deaths of 3%
- programme C increased the rate of survival from 84% to 87%
- programme D meant that 31 people needed to receive coronary rehab to prevent one death.

These were, of course, equivalent descriptions of one and the same outcome of an actual randomised trial in which these two treatments were compared. You might think that in deciding which programme to fund, this informed group would not have been influenced by the differences in presentation – but they were. The managers saw programme A as having the greatest merit and were most willing to fund where the benefits were expressed in terms of relative risk. Only three of the 140 managers realised that all four figures reflected the same clinical results.

We can be persuasive with information. Pharmaceutical companies use powerful techniques to present effects of their drugs to professionals. A survey of the leaflets for patients on mammography found that to encourage uptake, only information on relative risk was presented. As we have seen, this format is more 'effective' (Slaytor and Ward 1998). Perhaps this presentational selection is justifiable in some situations, to achieve the greatest public health gain, but presenting information in such a way is not consistent with truly informed decision-making. The effects of different ways of presenting information are summarised in Box 1.7 (Edwards, *et al.* 2002).

BOX 1.7 The effects of framing and other manipulations

- Information on relative risk is more persuasive than absolute risk data.
- 'Loss' framing (e.g. the potential losses from not having a mammogram) influences screening uptake more than 'gain' framing.
- Positive framing (e.g. chance of survival) is more effective than negative framing (e.g. chance of death) in persuading people to take risky options, such as treatments.
- More information, and information that is more understandable to the patient, is associated with a greater wariness to take treatments or tests.

(Edwards, *et al.* 2002)

PRINCIPLES FOR FUTURE COMMUNICATION OF RISKS (EDWARDS, *ET AL.* 2002)

- *Information should be simple and balanced.* Comparison with 'everyday risks' with which people are familiar may help to present risk data. Information on relative risk should not be presented in isolation. It seems sensible to employ both absolute and relative risk formats. The former include the number needed to treat and the number needed to harm, but these can be hard to interpret.
- *Risk information relevant to individuals is more valuable than average population data.* For example, an individual's risk of future coronary heart disease can be calculated by using information on risk factors (such as age, hypertension, cholesterol, smoking status or diabetes) from readily available charts.
- *Information must be presented clearly.* Sometimes numerical data alone may suffice. The visual presentation of risk information has also been explored. Some studies suggest that many patients prefer simple bar charts to other formats such as thermometer scales, crowd figures (e.g. showing how many in a group of 100 people are affected), survival curves or pie charts (Lipkus and Hollands 1999).
- *Most patients express a strong desire for information, but care is required to avoid overloading them.* In this regard, two major strengths of general practice are (1) that information can be provided in the light of the doctor's knowledge of the patient and his or her family and (2) that information can be discussed over several consultations.

In summary, health professionals need to be aware of their patients' need for information, be clear what their own views are and how they may colour what they say, be practised in the use of language and the tools they use, and be versatile in their application in differing circumstances.

CONCLUSION

Patients and the public are rightly demanding a greater voice in judging and improving quality. This greater level of involvement will require further research on what outcomes matter to patients and action on how best to meaningfully involve the public. It will also require new structures at national and local levels of provider and commissioning organisations for greater involvement. Finally, it will require training and resources for patients, carers and public representatives (NHS England 2013).

BOX 1.8 Resources for patients – databases and websites that practitioners can refer patients to

- HealthTalkOnline (http://healthtalkonline.org), originally the Database of Individual Patient Experiences, contains patients' experiences, including narratives of decision pathways.
- The UK National Library for Health (www.library.nhs.uk) includes different levels of information for patients.
- NHS Choices (www.nhs.uk/) is a website providing information and advice on illness and well-being.
- Health Crossroads (www.healthcrossroads.com) has audio overviews for over 70 decisions (or 'crossroads') in different conditions including breast cancer, benign uterine conditions (such as fibroids), prostate disease, coronary artery disease and back pain.

BOX 1.9 Prehospital emergency pain management

Pain management in emergency care is an important aspect of quality. A qualitative study with interviews and focus groups of patients, ambulance and emergency department staff helped us to understand their experiences during the patient pathway for emergency management of pain and how this could be improved.

Although patients and healthcare staff expected pain to be relieved in the ambulance, refusal of analgesia or acceptance of inadequate analgesia occurred because patients feared adverse drug effects, were loath to be transported, or were concerned that pain relief (e.g. with drugs such as morphine) would interfere with subsequent hospital assessment. Patients and practitioners found pain scores confusing. When clinical observations of staff disagreed with patient-reported pain scores, practitioners often responded according to presumed diagnosis rather than the patient's pain severity leading to over- or under-treatment.

Barriers to assessment of pain included communication difficulties or lack of cooperation due to the influence of alcohol or drugs. Morphine and Entonox were commonly used to treat pain, but reassurance, positioning and immobilisation were often used as alternatives to drugs.

Suggestions to improve prehospital pain management included addressing identified barriers, increasing drug options and developing agreed multi-organisational pain management protocols with appropriate training for staff.

This has led to further work to develop a patient-reported outcome measure for prehospital pain management.

(Iqbal, *et al.* 2013)

FURTHER READING

- Balestracci D (2009) The ins and outs of surveys: understanding the customer. In: Balestracci D Jr (ed). *Data sanity: a quantum leap to unprecedented results.* Medical Group Management Association: Englewood. pp. 269–80.
- Wensing M, Elwyn G (2004) Research on patients' views in the evaluation and improvement of quality of care. In: Grol R, Baker RH, Moss F (eds). *Quality improvement research: understanding the science of change in health care.* BMJ Books: London. pp. 64–77.

REFERENCES

Balint M (1957) *The doctor, his patient and the illness.* Pitman: London.

Barr M, Ginsburg J (2006) *The advanced medical home: a patient-centred, physician-guided model of health care.* American College of Physicians: Philadelphia, PA.

Black N, Jenkinson C (2009) Measuring patients' experiences and outcomes. *BMJ.* **339**: b2495.

Budescu DV, Weinberg S, Wallsten TS (1988) Decisions based on numerically and verbally expressed uncertainties. *J Exp Psychol Gen.* **14**: 281–94.

Carter M, Roland M, Campbell J, *et al.* (2009) *Using the GP Patient Survey to improve patient care: a guide for general practices.* National Primary Care Research and Development Centre: Manchester.

Coulter A, Locock L, Ziebland S, *et al.* (2014) Collecting data on patient experience is not enough: they must be used to improve care. *BMJ.* **348**: g2225.

Darzi of Denham AD (2008) *High quality care for all: NHS Next Stage Review final report.* CM 7432. The Stationery Office: London.

De Silva D (2013) *Measuring patient experience.* Evidence scan No. 18. The Health Foundation: London.

Deming WE (1982) *Out of the crisis.* Massachusetts Institute of Technology, Center for Advanced Engineering Study: Cambridge, MA.

Department of Health (2011) *NHS Patient Experience Framework.* Department of Health: London.

Department of Health (2013a) *The NHS Constitution for England: the NHS belongs to us all.* Department of Health: London.

Department of Health (2013b) *The NHS Outcomes Framework 2014/15.* Williams Lea: London.

Department of Health (2010) *Equity and excellence: liberating the NHS.* The Stationery Office: Norwich.

Doyle C, Lennox L, Bell D (2013) A systematic review of evidence on the links between patient experience and clinical safety and effectiveness. *BMJ Open.* **3**(1): e001570.

Dyas JV, Apekey TA, Tilling M, *et al.* (2010) Patients' and clinicians' experiences of consultations in primary care for sleep problems and insomnia: a focus group study. *Br J Gen Pract.* **60**(574): 180–200.

Edwards A, Elwyn G, Mulley A. (2002) Explaining risks: turning numerical data into meaningful pictures. *BMJ.* **324**(7341): 827–30.

Edwards A, Hood K, Matthews E, *et al.* (2000) The effectiveness of one-to-one risk communication interventions in health care: a systematic review. *Med Decis Making.* **20**(3): 290–7.

Fahey T, Griffiths S, Peters TJ (1995) Evidence based purchasing: understanding results of clinical trials and systematic reviews. *BMJ.* **311**(7012): 1056–9.

Francis R (2010) *Robert Francis inquiry report into Mid-Staffordshire NHS Foundation Trust.* The Stationery Office: London.

Gillam S, Siriwardena AN (2010) *The Quality and Outcomes Framework: QOF transforming general practice.* Radcliffe Publishing: Oxford.

Guthrie B, Saultz JW, Freeman GK, *et al.* (2008) Continuity of care matters. *BMJ.* **337**: a867.

Guthrie B, Wyke S (2006) Access and continuity in UK general practice: a qualitative study of general practitioners' and patients' perceptions of when and how they matter. *BMC Fam Pract.* 7: 11.

Haggerty JL, Reid RJ, Freeman GK, *et al.* (2003) Continuity of care: a multidisciplinary review. *BMJ.* **327**(7425): 1219–21.

Institute of Medicine (2001) *Crossing the quality chasm: a new health system for the 21st century.* The National Academies Press: Washington, DC.

Iqbal M, Spaight PA, Siriwardena AN (2013) Patients' and emergency clinicians' perceptions of improving pre-hospital pain management: a qualitative study. *Emerg Med J.* 30(3): e18.

Juran JM, Godfrey AB (1999) *Juran's quality handbook.* McGraw Hill: New York, NY.

Kahneman D (2012) *Thinking, fast and slow.* Penguin: London.

Keogh B (2013) *Review into the quality of care and treatment provided by 14 hospital trusts in England: overview report.* Department of Health: London.

Lipkus IM, Hollands JG (1999) The visual communication of risk. *J Natl Cancer Inst Monogr.* (25): 149–63.

Nagraj S, Gillam S (2011) Patient participation groups. *BMJ.* **342**: d2333.

National Advisory Group on the Safety of Patients in England (2013) *A promise to learn – a commitment to act: improving the safety of patients in England.* National Advisory Group on the Safety of Patients in England: London.

National Institute for Health and Clinical Excellence (2012) *Patient experience in adult NHS services: improving the experience of care for people using adult NHS services.* Clinical guideline 138. NICE: Manchester.

NHS England (2013) *Transforming participation in health and care: 'The NHS belongs to us all'.* Patients and Information Directorate, NHS England: London.

NHS Information Centre (2011) *General Practice Bulletin, 2000–2010.* 22 March.

Saultz JW, Albedaiwi W (2004) Interpersonal continuity of care and patient satisfaction: a critical review. *Ann Fam Med.* 2(5): 445–51.

Sequist TD, Schneider EC, Anastario M, *et al.* (2008) Quality monitoring of physicians: linking patients' experiences of care to clinical quality and outcomes. *J Gen Intern Med.* 23(11): 1784–90.

Siriwardena AN (2014) *Assessment and management of insomnia e-learning package. Resources for Effective Sleep Treatment.* University of Lincoln: Lincoln.

Siriwardena AN, Norfolk T (2007) The enigma of patient centredness, the therapeutic relationship and outcomes of the clinical encounter. *Qual Prim Care.* 15: 1–4.

Slaytor EK, Ward JE (1998) How risks of breast cancer and benefits of screening are communicated to women: analysis of 58 pamphlets. *BMJ.* 317(7152): 263–4.

Wiig S, Storm M, Aase K, *et al.* (2013) Investigating the use of patient involvement and patient experience in quality improvement in Norway: rhetoric or reality? *BMC Health Serv Res.* **13**: 206.

Williamson C (2007) 'How do we find the right patients to consult?' *Qual Prim Care.* 15: 195–9.

CHAPTER 2

Leadership and management

SUMMARY

- Leadership and management skills are integral to the successful delivery of quality improvement initiatives.
- Management can be considered in terms of principles, theories, structures, behaviours and techniques.
- Effective leaders adapt their style to the needs of their team, the task and the characteristics of their organisation.
- An understanding of the factors that influence behaviour is as important for achieving change within organisations as it is for helping individuals.

INTRODUCTION

Management in healthcare is about getting things done to improve the care of patients. Leadership skills help doctors become more actively involved in planning and delivery of health services and also in support roles in research, education and health politics. Management competencies are crucially important to health professionals for ensuring systems are in place to monitor and maintain quality of care: the stuff of 'clinical governance' and the focus of this series.

THE NATURE OF MANAGEMENT

Classical management theories evolved out of military theory and were developed further as advanced societies industrialised. While they recognised the need to harmonise human aspects of the organisation, problems were essentially seen as technical. Early theories made individuals fit the requirements of the organisation. Later theories borrowing on behavioural psychology and sociology suggest ways in which the organisation needs to fit the requirements of individuals.

Point to ponder
- What do you think managers do?

Most front-line practitioners work closely alongside managers, understand what they actually do, and can therefore see them as partners in improving patient care.

We can think about management in terms of the tasks or actions a manager needs to perform (*see* Box 2.1), but it is also useful to think of management as having several different dimensions, as follows (Gillam and Klein 2001).

- **Principles:** management is about people, securing commitment to shared values, developing staff and achieving results. These help determine the culture of organisations.
- **Theories:** management is underpinned by a plethora of different theories and frameworks. These, in turn, shape the language – and jargon – of management.
- **Structures:** the way organisations are set up (e.g. as bureaucracies, open systems, matrices, networks).
- **Behaviours:** personal and organisational.
- **Techniques:** including communication skills, management by objectives, finance, accounting, planning, marketing, project management and quality assurance.

BOX 2.1 Management tasks

- **Defining the task:** break down general aims into specific manageable tasks.
- **Planning:** be creative – think laterally and use the ideas of others. Evaluate the options and formulate a working plan. Turn a negative situation into a positive one by creative planning.
- **Briefing:** communicate the plan. Run meetings, make presentations and write clear instructions. The five skills of briefing are Preparing, Clarifying, Simplifying, Vivifying (making the subject alive), Being yourself.
- **Controlling:** work out what key facts need to be monitored to see if the plan is working, and set standards to measure them against. To control others, you need also to be able to control yourself (e.g. managing your time to best effect).
- **Evaluating:** assess the consequences of your efforts. Some form of progress report and/or debriefing meeting will enable people to see what they are achieving. The people as well as the task need evaluating, and the techniques of appraisal are important tasks for the leader of the team.
- **Motivating:** simple ways often work best. Recognition, for instance, of someone's efforts, be it by promotion, extra money or, more frequently, by personal commendation, seldom fails. Success motivates people and communicates a new sense of energy and urgency to the group.
- **Organising:** see that the infrastructure for the work is in place and operating effectively.
- **Setting an example:** research on successful organisations suggests that key factors are the behaviour, the values and the standards of their leaders. People take more notice of what you are and what you do than what you say.
- **Communicating:** be clear and focused. Who needs to know what in order to get your aims realised?
- **Housekeeping:** manage yourself – your time and other resources. Have coping strategies for recognising and dealing with pressure for yourself and others.

THEORIES OF LEADERSHIP

There are various theories of leadership. Early writers tended to suggest that leaders were born not made, but no one has been able to agree on a particular set of characteristics required.

The following are commonly listed as leadership qualities:
- above average intelligence
- initiative or the capacity to perceive the need for action and do something about it
- self-assurance, courage and integrity
- being able to rise above a particular situation and see it in its broader context (the 'helicopter trait')
- high energy levels
- high achievement career-wise
- being goal directed and being able to think longer term
- good communication skills and the ability to work with a wide variety of people.

Modern theories have proposed two types of leadership: transactional and transformational. Transactional leadership attempts to preserve the status quo, while transformational leadership seeks to inspire and engage the emotions of individuals in organisations. Transactional leadership concentrates on exchanges between leaders and staff, offering rewards for meeting particular standards in performance. Transformational leadership highlights the importance of leaders demonstrating inspirational motivation and concentrates on relationships (Bennis and Nanus 2003). Another popular concept to emerge in more recent literature on leadership is that of 'emotional intelligence' (Goleman 1996). This is the capacity for recognising our own feelings and those of others, motivating ourselves and managing emotions well in ourselves.

> **Point to ponder**
> - What qualities characterise the leaders you have encountered?

Note that leadership and management are not synonymous. A manager is an individual who holds an office to which roles are attached, whereas leadership is one of the roles attached to the office of manager. Just being in a senior position will not make you a leader, and certainly not an influential one. Both leaders and managers wield power and must have the ability to influence others to achieve organisational aims (*see* Box 2.2).

How you carry out your managerial functions and the way you exercise power and authority – your management and leadership style – is central. To be successful, it must be appropriate to the situation. Different styles are needed at different times and in different organisational contexts. All of us have preferred styles conditioned by personality and experience. The ability to adapt your approach to different circumstances is a major determinant of effectiveness, just as communication skills with individual patients require versatility according to circumstances.

In healthcare, increasing consideration is being given to the organisational context within which people work and what is required of a leader in that work

---

BOX 2.2 Sources of power

Power based on the position of the individual	Power based on the individual	Power based on the individual
Positional power Vested in an individual by virtue of the position they hold (e.g. 'team leader')		
	Expert power Specialist expertise such as that of an NHS consultant	***Personal power*** What an individual brings personally, such as style, charisma and skills
Resource power Control over staff, funds or other resources		

---

situation. According to contingency theories of leadership, four variables have to be taken into account when analysing different circumstances:

1 the manager (or leader) – his or her personality and preferred style
2 the managed (or led) – the needs, attitudes and skills of his or her subordinates or colleagues
3 the task – requirements and goals of the job to be done
4 the context – the organisation and its values and prejudices.

Unsurprisingly, the one over which you have most control is you!

THEORIES OF CHANGE

Surveying most health systems, two features are immediately apparent. The first is their extraordinary complexity as ever more sophisticated technology is developed to meet an ever-expanding range of health problems. A second feature of modern healthcare is how fast new technologies and services are evolving. Leaders and managers in this environment are therefore concerned with understanding the need for and managing change.

Lewin (1947) developed the notion of 'force field analysis' to help understand drivers and barriers to change; reducing forces resisting change is considered to be more effective than strengthening driving forces, but it is important to address both. There are many management tools that can be used to analyse change and the forces that might support or hinder it. For example, a PESTLE analysis (Chartered Institute of Personnel and Development 2013) can be used to consider the context within which a specific change is occurring. PESTLE is an acronym covering the influences on an organisation (*see* Box 2.3).

Introducing a new service or changing an existing service in response to the kind of drivers identified by using a tool such as PESTLE is difficult. Many people will initially resist change, even if the results are likely to benefit them. The process of change involves helping people within an organisation or a system to change the way they work and interact with others in the system. Leaders need to understand how people respond to change in order to plan it.

BOX 2.3 PESTLE analysis

Political	**Environmental**	**Social**
What is happening politically that could affect your organisation? (E.g. government policy)	What environmental issues affect your organisation? (E.g. carbon reduction requirements)	How do social factors affect your organisation? (E.g. population growth, ageing)

Technological	**Legal**	**Economic**
How does changing technology affect your organisation? (E.g. new drugs, medical devices)	What legal factors influence your organisation? (E.g. medico-legal requirements, registration)	What are the implications of finances and economics on your organisation? (E.g. taxes, payment models)

Point to ponder
- Think about your organisation or a healthcare system. You could use the whole of the National Health Service (NHS). Use the PESTLE model to analyse what is driving change in that system.

Everett Rogers's classic model (*see* Figure 2.1) of how people take up an innovation can help us to understand different people's responses to change (Rogers 2003). This was originally based on observations of how farmers took up hybrid seed corn in Iowa. The model describes the differential rate of uptake of an innovation, in order to target promotion of the product, and labels people according to their place on the uptake curve. Rogers's original model described the 'late adopters' as 'laggards', but this seems a pejorative term when there may be good reasons not to take up the innovation. How soon after their introduction, for example, should nurses and doctors be prescribing new, usually more expensive, inhalers for asthma?

Individuals' 'change type' may depend on the particular change they are adopting. This depends on the perceived benefits, the perceived obstacles and the motivation to make the change.

People are more likely to adopt an innovation:
- that provides a **relative advantage** compared with old ideas
- that is **compatible** with the existing value system of the adopter
- that is readily understood by the adopters (**less complexity**)
- where the results of the innovation are more easily noticed by other potential adopters (**observability**).

Pharmaceutical companies use this model in their approaches to general practitioners (GPs). The local sales representatives know from the information they have about GPs in their area whether a GP is an early adopter. Early adopters are often opinion leaders in a community. Early on in the process of promotion, sales representatives will target those GPs with personal visits, whereas they may send the late adopters an information leaflet only, as those GPs will

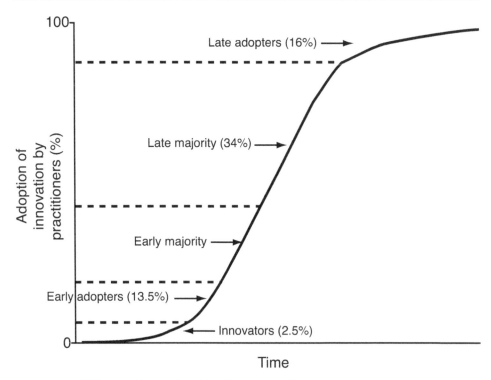

FIGURE 2.1 Diffusion of innovation (after Rogers 2003)

not consider change until more than 80% of their colleagues have taken up the new product.

Clinicians will be familiar with other psychological models of change from their 'day jobs'. For example, the transtheoretical model describes the process of behaviour change in terms of different motivational states during adoption of an innovation (Prochaska and Diclemente 1983).

The process begins with precontemplation (not yet ready for change) and progresses through contemplation (thinking about change), preparation (for change), action (to implement change) and finally maintenance of change. The skills required to motivate individual behavioural change overlap with those required at an organisational level.

ORGANISATIONAL BEHAVIOUR AND MOTIVATION
It is important to understand how people operate within the organisation within which they work. Organisational behaviour can be studied at three levels: in relation to (1) individuals, (2) teams and (3) organisational processes (Robbins and Judge 2007). Managers everywhere are interested in how such concepts as job satisfaction, commitment, motivation and team dynamics may increase productivity, innovation and competitiveness.

Types of organisation
How organisations function is a combination of their culture and structures. Organisational culture has been described as a set of norms, beliefs, principles

and ways of behaving that together give each organisation a distinctive character (Brown 1998). Handy describes four types of organisational culture (Box 2.4) which are dependent on power, role, task or person (Handy 1999).

BOX 2.4 Handy's types of organisational culture

Power culture

Power is held by a few and radiates out from the centre like a web

Few rules and bureaucracy mean that decisions can be swift

Role culture

Hierarchical bureaucracy where power derives from a person's position

Task culture

Power derives from expertise and structures are often matrix with teams forming as necessary

Person culture

All individuals are equal and operate collaboratively to pursue the organisational goals

---

Point to ponder
- In what type of organisation do you think you work? How does this influence your ability to do your job?

There is as yet limited evidence linking organisational culture and performance in primary care (Hann, *et al.* 2007). Great methodological ingenuity will be required to unravel the relationship between these two variables (Scott, *et al.* 2003).

Point to ponder
- What factors affect the behaviour of staff and teams in your workplace?

Types of team

Even relatively small organisations such as general practices may at some point form different types of team to carry our specific functions. Teams are often described as follows.

- **Vertical or functional.** Teams that carry out one function within an organisation, such as an infection control team within a practice or hospital.
- **Horizontal or cross-functional.** Teams that are made up of members from across an organisation. These may be formed for specific projects, such as managing the introduction of a new service which might need operational, clinical and financial input, or can be long-standing teams, such as an executive team running an organisation.
- **Self-directed.** Teams that do not have dedicated leadership or management. These may generate themselves within an organisation

to achieve aims or they can be specifically designed to give employees a feeling of ownership.

Tuckman's model (*see* Figure 2.2) explains how teams develop over time and can be used to consider how individuals, including the leader, behave within those teams (Tuckman 1965).

Getting the right people on the team is critical to a successful improvement effort. Teams vary in size and composition; each organisation builds teams to suit its own needs. Effective teams include members representing three different kinds of expertise within the organisation: (1) system leadership, (2) technical expertise and (3) day-to-day leadership.

LEADING CHANGE IN CLINICAL PRACTICE

We have described a number of theories relating to management, leadership and change. But how can these be used in clinical practice? Nowadays, clinicians increasingly occupy leadership positions, whether in general practices, hospitals, commissioning groups or regulatory agencies, exercising power with increasing managerial accountability for outcomes. They drive the changes that

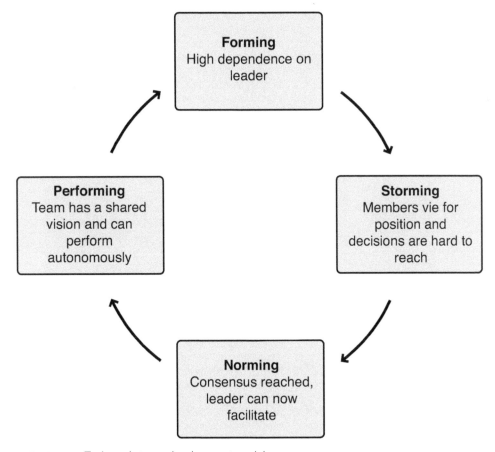

FIGURE 2.2 Tuckman's team development model

they believe – on the basis of evidence and experience – will result in improved health for their setting or population. Strategy is at the heart of the change process. Leadership and management skills are central to developing strategy for quality improvement (*see* Box 2.5).

Point to ponder
- How much do you think you will need achievement, power and affiliation in your future work?

BOX 2.5 Strategy development for quality improvement

How do we make the case for change?	• Assess local needs, taking account of national strategies • Define the drivers for and against change (e.g. through PESTLE analysis)
What are we aiming to do?	• Clarify aims, objectives and desired outcomes • Define local standards and set targets
How can we make change happen?	• Understand the principles of change management and plan to address the factors that might resist change • Include a description of the actions that are required, and an assessment of the resource implications of putting the new service into place with clear financial plans • Consider the organisational context and how you need teams and individuals to operate in the new system
How do we engage with partners including patients?	• Involve all those who are affected by the strategy including clinicians, managers and other staff in and in partner organisations • Identify who will support and who will oppose it; develop an approach to overcoming this opposition; consider who has the power in these relationships and how that affects the strategy development
How do we know we have done what we wanted to do?	• Evaluate impact by demonstrating achievement against the standards and targets through monitoring routine data and special studies
How do we make successful change become normal practice?	• The change in practice needs to be sustained to ensure that it becomes routine, as people tend to revert to their old ways of working • This requires individuals to change the way they do things; continuing education and alterations to the work environment with a process of ongoing monitoring/audit/feedback may all be required • Consider what motivates people and how to use leadership and management skills to build a culture of continuous improvement

NHS Improving Quality was established in 2013 to drive improvement across the NHS by building capacity, improving knowledge and skills (NHS IQ 2014). The current reforms to the NHS highlight the role of clinicians, especially doctors, as both leaders and managers. The UK Leadership Council's NHS Leadership Framework is built on a concept of shared leadership and sets out the competencies doctors and other NHS professionals need to run healthcare organisations and improve quality of care (Academy of Medical Royal Colleges and NHS Institute for Innovation and Improvement 2010). The domains of this framework are shown in Figure 2.3.

Such competencies in leadership and management develop over an individual's career. Leadership and management behaviours can be learned, but continuous improvement requires an open-minded approach to assessing our own skills level, an ability to seek and accept constructive feedback on our performance and a willingness to change. How can we lead and manage change if we are unwilling to lead, manage and change ourselves?

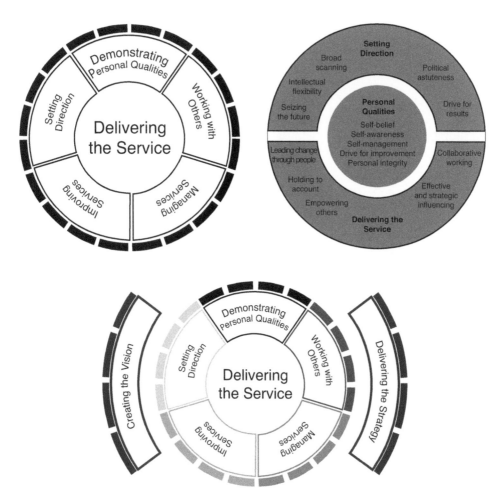

FIGURE 2.3 The UK NHS Leadership Framework

Point to ponder
- Think of a new service or change, large or small, that would require leadership and management to deliver. Use the questions in Box 2.5 and the theory outlined in this chapter to consider how you would go about managing that change.

REFERENCES

Academy of Medical Royal Colleges, NHS Institute for Innovation and Improvement (2010) *Medical Leadership Competency Framework: enhancing engagement in medical leadership*. NHS Institute for Innovation and Improvement, University of Warwick: Coventry.

Bennis WG, Nanus B (2003) *Leaders: strategies for taking charge*. Harper Business Essentials: New York, NY.

Brown AD (1998) *Organisational culture*. Financial Times/Pitman: London.

Chartered Institute of Personnel and Development (2013) *PESTLE analysis factsheet*. CIPD: London.

Gillam S, Klein R (2001) *What has New Labour done for primary care? A balance sheet*. The King's Fund: London.

Goleman D (1996) *Emotional intelligence: why it can matter more than IQ*. Bloomsbury: London.

Handy CB (1999). *Understanding organizations*, 4th ed. Penguin: London.

Hann M, Bower P, Campbell S, *et al.* (2007) The association between culture, climate and quality of care in primary health care teams. *Fam Pract.* 24(4): 323–9.

Lewin K (1947) Frontiers in group dynamics. *Hum Relat.* 1: 4–41.

NHS Improving Quality (2014) An introduction to NHS Improving Quality. www.nhsiq. nhs.uk/resource-search/publications/intro-to-nhs-iq.aspx

Prochaska JO, Diclemente CC (1983) Stages and processes of self-change of smoking: toward an integrative model of change. *J Consult Clin Psychol.* 51(3): 390–5.

Robbins SP, Judge T (2007) *Organizational behavior*. Pearson/Prentice Hall: Upper Saddle River, NJ.

Rogers EM (2003) *Diffusion of innovations*. 5th ed. Free Press: New York, NY.

Scott T, Mannion R, Marshall M, *et al.* (2003) Does organisational culture influence health care performance? A review of the evidence. *J Health Serv Res Policy.* 8(2): 105–17.

Tuckman BW (1965) Developmental sequence in small groups. *Psychol Bull.* 63: 384–99.

CHAPTER 3

Regulation

SUMMARY

- Professional bodies have long overseen the maintenance of standards of training and practice within the different healthcare professions, but in recent years, the role of government has increased.
- Organisational regulation of healthcare in England comprises two main elements: (1) regulation of the quality and safety of care offered by healthcare providers, currently undertaken by the Care Quality Commission (CQC), and (2) regulation of the market in healthcare services, currently the responsibility of Monitor and the Department of Health.
- Various bodies operate at different levels to protect the public, improve quality of care and achieve greater value for money. The cost-effectiveness of these new arrangements is unknown – and possibly unknowable.
- New forms of governance and regulation encouraging collaboration and partnership between a wider range of professional and public stakeholders may provide greater opportunities for quality improvement.

INTRODUCTION

All health professionals work in healthcare systems that are regulated by professional bodies and government organisations. With 1.7 million employees and an annual budget of £104 billion, the National Health Service (NHS) is one of the largest organisations in the world and there are complex regulatory structures in place that aim to ensure that patients receive high-quality care. Despite this, adverse events can (and do) occur. Government-led investigations such as the Shipman and Mid Staffordshire inquiries have sadly served to remind us that organisational failings and the actions of individuals can place patients at risk. A challenge for successive governments has been to develop systems that regulate healthcare professionals and the organisations in which they work, to ensure that the public are protected, and quality of care is enhanced while achieving greater value for money (Department of Health 2007; Allsop and Saks 2008).

PROFESSIONAL REGULATORS

Currently, regulation in healthcare occurs on many different levels. Individual healthcare practitioners, such as doctors, nurses and allied health professionals, are required by law to apply for licences to practise from their professional regulators (e.g. the General Medical Council, or GMC), of which there are nine in the United Kingdom (*see* Box 3.1).

Regulators determine the qualifications required for licensing, maintain professional registers, provide codes of practice and ethics to members, investigate more serious complaints about individual practice and discipline those who fail to meet standards set (Allsop and Saks 2002).

Over 1.3 million professionals carrying out 32 different roles hold such licences, and the performance of their regulators is overseen by the Professional Standards Authority for Health and Social Care. This aims to review and harmonise the activities of the different professional bodies through regular reviews and reports to parliament via the Health Committee.

BOX 3.1 The nine UK regulators and the professions they regulate

1   General Chiropractic Council (GCC) – regulates chiropractors
2   General Dental Council (GDC) – regulates dentists, dental nurses, dental technicians, dental hygienists, dental therapists, clinical dental technicians and orthodontic therapists
3   General Medical Council (GMC) – regulates doctors
4   General Optical Council (GOC) – regulates optometrists and dispensing opticians
5   General Osteopathic Council (GOsC) – regulates osteopaths
6   General Pharmaceutical Council (GPhC) – regulates pharmacists and pharmacy technicians
7   Health and Care Professions Council (HCPC) – regulates arts therapists, biomedical scientists, chiropodists/podiatrists, clinical scientists, dieticians, hearing aid dispensers, occupational therapists, operating department practitioners, orthoptists, paramedics, physiotherapists, practitioner psychologists, prosthetists/orthotists, radiographers, social workers, and speech and language therapists
8   Nursing and Midwifery Council (NMC) – regulates nurses and midwives
9   Pharmaceutical Society of Northern Ireland (PSNI) – regulates pharmacists

---

The GMC was created 'to protect, promote, and maintain the health and safety of the public by ensuring proper standards in the practice of medicine' (General Medical Council 2014) and is currently adapting to a new environment where greater levels of public accountability are required. As set out in the Medical Act 1983, its main role is to keep a register of qualified doctors and erase from the register those who are deemed unfit to practise. However, this role has evolved over the past decade or so and the GMC is now also responsible for setting standards in medical education and professional conduct, and for periodic revalidation.

Revalidation is the process by which all licensed doctors are required to demonstrate once every five years that they are up to date and fit to practise. It aims to give extra confidence to patients that their doctor's professional knowledge is up to date. Doctors are assessed using their annual appraisals and supporting portfolios (Chambers 2008). The GMC expects to revalidate the majority of licensed doctors in the United Kingdom for the first time by March 2016.

Established in 2002, the Nursing and Midwifery Council (NMC) is the UK regulator for nursing and midwifery professions. The NMC maintains a register of all nurses, midwives and specialist community public health nurses eligible to practise within the United Kingdom. It sets and reviews standards for their education, training, conduct and performance. The NMC also investigates allegations of impaired fitness to practise where these standards are not met. Nurses should be appraised annually via their employers, although a comparable system of revalidation is not yet compulsory. Indeed, little is known of the extent to which nurses are currently being appraised within general practice.

The Health and Care Professions Council, which regulates allied health, psychological and social work professionals, will become an increasingly important player in the regulatory landscape with changes in the health and social care workforce that affect skill mix as part of service improvement and redesign (Butterworth 2008).

> **Point to ponder**
> ● What activities and features of your professional regulator are conducive to quality improvement?

ORGANISATIONAL REGULATION

Responsibilities for regulating 'organisational' rather than 'individual' aspects of healthcare delivery in England, Scotland and Wales are split across different bodies (*see* Box 3.2) with varying powers, roles and remits.

BOX 3.2 Healthcare regulators in the United Kingdom

England
● Care Quality Commission (CQC)
● Monitor

Scotland
● Healthcare Improvement Scotland
● Care Inspectorate

Wales
● Care and Social Services Inspectorate Wales
● Healthcare Inspectorate Wales

In 1997, there was no national policy covering all aspects of safety and quality of healthcare provision. The New Labour government concluded that the quality of care provided by the NHS had been 'variable' and that the service had been slow to respond to 'serious lapses in quality', notably at the Bristol Royal Infirmary (Department of Health 1997).

The Commission for Healthcare Improvement was established in 1999 to offer guidance to NHS providers on clinical governance. The Healthcare Commission was established in 2003 to bring together the work of Commission for Healthcare Improvement, the National Standards Commission (the independent regulatory body responsible for inspecting and regulating residential and domiciliary care) and also the value-for-money activity relating to the NHS that was carried out by the Audit Commission.

Pressure to reduce the number of regulators led to the establishment of the Care Quality Commission (CQC) in 2009. This brought together the Healthcare Commission, the Commission for Social Care Inspection and the Mental Health Act Commission. The CQC regulates and inspects the quality and safety of all providers of healthcare and adult social care services. It registers and scrutinises hospitals, ambulance services, clinics, community services, care homes, mental health services, dental practices and, since April 2012, general practices.

Registration requirements cover areas such as the management and training of staff, the state of premises and provision of information. Using information from a wide range of sources, the CQC focuses on outcomes for service users and has a wide range of enforcement powers, including closure and deregistration of services, if essential standards are not met.

Recent scandals, notably at the Mid Staffordshire NHS Foundation Trust, highlighted major deficiencies in the CQC's hospital inspection regimen but wholesale reorganisation has been favourably received (Dyer 2014). How successfully it has addressed deficiencies in general practice is as yet unknown.

NHS organisations are also subject to oversight by many other regulators with a specific health remit, such as the Medicines and Healthcare Products Regulatory Agency (MHRA), the Health and Safety Executive responsible for employee health and safety, or the Human Fertilisation and Embryology Authority, which licenses fertility clinics and human embryo research.

The MHRA was established in 2003 as an agency of the Department of Health to protect the public through the regulation of medicines, medical devices and equipment used in healthcare. Any product used for the diagnosis, prevention, monitoring or treatment of illness or disability is classed as a medical device. The MHRA monitors the many thousands of items used every day by professionals and patients, ranging from contact lenses and walking sticks through to heart valves, computerised tomography scanners and defibrillators.

MARKET REGULATION

Some NHS services have always been provided by private sector bodies – most general practitioners are in fact independent contractors, operating as small businesses contracted to provide NHS services but also delivering non-NHS services. Successive governments, however, actively promoted an expansion of private provision of hospital and community services, with the aim of creating a mixed economy in which any willing – and licensed – provider could offer services to NHS patients. Patients, or commissioners acting on their behalf, have been free to choose where to go for treatment.

This led to new forms of regulation to ensure that market forces worked to the benefit of patients. For example, allowing patients to choose where they received hospital treatment required a new hospital payment system that reimburses hospitals for the number of patients treated and the types of treatment given. The Department of Health sets a national tariff for most hospital activity, to encourage competition on the basis of quality of service, rather than cost.

The Co-operation and Competition Panel was established to offer advice to ministers on mergers of NHS bodies – as these could reduce the extent of competition – and to monitor how commissioners adhere to rules on when to tender for services. Private sector providers can appeal to the panel if they feel they have not been given a fair opportunity to compete.

MONITOR

To strengthen the ability of NHS providers to respond to market opportunities, the government introduced a new form of NHS organisation, the foundation trust. These enjoyed greater financial freedoms and less direct control by the Secretary of State than traditional NHS trusts. In 2004, a new regulator, Monitor, was established in England to vet applications for foundation trust status and to oversee their financial performance once they were in operation.

The coalition government's Health and Social Care Act 2012 made significant changes to Monitor's role. Since April 2013 it has become *the* sector regulator for healthcare, with responsibility for regulating and licensing all providers of NHS-funded services. Monitor's stated aim is to:

> protect and promote the interests of people who use health care services by promoting the provision of services which are economic, efficient and effective, and to maintain or improve the quality of the services.

Monitor sets the tariff for NHS-funded services and works with the NHS England – a new organisation set up to carry out some national commissioning functions – to develop tariffs and prices. The Co-operation and Competition Panel has been absorbed into Monitor, but eventually the NHS will come within the remit of the Office of Fair Trading and be subject to European Union competition law.

The coalition government has proposed greater freedom for foundation trusts – for example, in respect of their governance arrangements, their ability to raise capital and their ability to raise income from private patients. Monitor has responsibility for continuity of essential trust services – for example, in the event of financial failure. These proposals are thus designed to take the development of a mixed economy of provision further, and so extend the scope of the independent regulators and consequently reduce that of the Department of Health.

DOES REGULATION 'WORK'?

There is little evidence to draw on to address this question. International comparisons are of limited value. The King's Fund reviewed regulation in four healthcare systems – New Zealand, Catalonia, Germany and the Netherlands – all of which have similarities with the English NHS. All five countries have to regulate a healthcare system comprising public, for-profit and not-for-profit independent providers. Although these health systems have many similar objectives to the NHS, there is no agreement on the best way to regulate healthcare systems, and regulation must be appropriate to the particular structure of each system (Lewis, *et al.* 2006).

The regulatory framework of healthcare in England is still developing – the government's proposals leave a number of questions unanswered. The boundaries between the different regulators, NHS England and the Secretary of State need clarification. What should be the objectives of the economic regulator and who should set them? If prices are to be set, who should do this? Should price competition be allowed? How should the tension between promoting cooperation, networking and integration and maintaining competition be resolved? How effectively will clinical commissioning groups be regulated?

There is some evidence that regulation may exert effects through potential reputational damage, loss or gain of organisational or personal kudos and risk to senior leaders' positions (Bevan and Hamblin 2009). Although this might be effective in achieving standards, this needs to be set against unintended consequences such as gaming, falsifying data or measurement fixation (Hamblin 2008).

Ultimately, it is important to ensure that the benefits accruing from the large bureaucratic organisations involved in regulation outweigh their costs. The United States provides a ghastly reminder of the potential burdens of this 'hidden tax'. Healthcare regulation may cost in excess of $500 billion and yield one-third as much in benefit (Conover 2004). Governments are trying to balance increased accountability of health services with improved quality and local innovation in service design and delivery while reducing the overall costs of regulation (Scrivens 2007), and governments are experimenting with risk-based approaches to achieve this (Adil 2008).

Increasingly, lay membership of professional and organisational regulatory bodies is being strengthened. Lay members bring the user and patient perspective to the fore in discussions and decisions of regulators, providing a viewpoint that is complementary to that of professionals. Finally, lay members add credibility to the regulatory framework (Ali 2008).

Point to ponder
- How can regulation work better to encourage quality improvement in the setting you work in?

REGULATION IN (GENERAL) PRACTICE

CQC registration is an arduous process but focuses on important practice systems (e.g. risk management, patient safety, information technology, maintenance, employment practice). The new Chief Inspector of General Practice is responsible for developing a framework for monitoring practices, which will further stretch administrative and clinical resources (Care Quality Commission 2013). It is easy to see these encroachments in entirely negative terms (Matthews-King 2013). The key for health professionals – as with individual appraisals – is to make the process work for you and your organisation.

This means using inspections and audit to identify and 'fix' areas for

improvement. If what is measured is what matters, teams will 'buy in' to procedures and help routinise data collection. Practice teams without strong
leadership or a clear vision of where they are going will struggle to adapt.
Against a backdrop of labour shortages, the next few years are likely to be testing for many general practices. However, constructive regulatory procedures
can help to improve patient care.

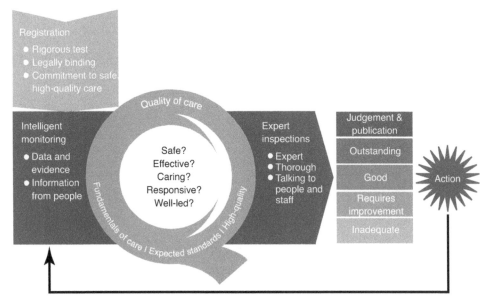

FIGURE 3.1 Overview of the Care Quality Commission's proposed operating model

Point to ponder
- How are you and your organisation preparing for your CQC inspection?

CONCLUSION

A robust regulatory framework is important for assuring a basic standard of
healthcare. The regulation of medical professionals and healthcare providers is
a central component of quality improvement in most countries. The NHS faces
the challenges of an ageing population, an increase in long-term conditions,
costly scientific and technological advances, and an unsustainable growth in
healthcare spending together with rising public expectations.

The recent restructuring of the health service and legislative changes give
regulatory organisations greatly increased powers over healthcare organisations including general practices. New forms of governance and regulation that
encourage collaboration and partnership between a wider range of professional
and public stakeholders provide opportunities for regulation to stimulate quality improvement rather than maintaining basic standards for care.

In addition, individual health professionals can expect their professional
practice to come under closer scrutiny as the process of revalidation is rolled out.

FURTHER READING

➡ Poulton B, Offredy M (2008) Professional regulation. Quality in Primary care. **16**: 223–67.

REFERENCES

Adil M (2008) Risk-based regulatory system and its effective use in health and social care. *J R Soc Promot Health*. **128**(4): 196–201.

Ali M (2008) The future shape of healthcare regulation and the role of lay members. *Qual Prim Care*. **16**(4): 259–62.

Allsop J, Saks M (2008) Professional regulation in primary care: the long road to quality improvement. *Qual Prim Care*. **16**(4): 225–8.

Allsop J, Saks M (2002) *Regulating the health professions*. Sage: London.

Bevan G, Hamblin R (2009) Hitting and missing targets by ambulance services for emergency calls: effects of different systems of performance measurement within the UK. *J R Stat Soc Ser A Stat Soc*. **172**(1): 161–90.

Butterworth T (2008) The practice and regulation of non-medical healthcare professionals in community-based and primary care: maintaining old landscapes or encouraging creativity? *Qual Prim Care*. **16**(4): 231–3.

Care Quality Commission (2013) *A fresh start for the regulation and inspection of GP practices and GP out-of-hours services*. CQC: London.

Chambers R (2008) Professional regulation in primary care: improving quality and safety . . . we hope. *Qual Prim Care*. **16**(4): 235–8.

Conover C (2004) *Health care regulation: a $169 billion hidden tax*. No. 527. Cato Institute: Washington, DC.

Department of Health (2007) *Trust, assurance and safety: the regulation of health professionals in the 21st century*. The Stationery Office: London.

Department of Health (1997) *The New NHS: modern, dependable*. The Stationery Office: London.

Dyer C (2014) After period of failure, NHS regulator is now fit for purpose, say MPs. *BMJ*. **348**: g434.

General Medical Council (2014) *Our role*. GMC: London www.gmc-uk.org/about/role. asp (accessed 19 June 2014).

Hamblin R (2008) Regulation, measurements and incentives. The experience in the US and UK: does context matter? *J R Soc Promot Health*. **128**(6): 291–8.

Lewis R, Alvarez-Rosete A, Mays N (2006) *How to regulate health care in England? An international perspective*. The King's Fund: London.

Matthews-King A (2013) CQC threatens to send 'OFSTED-style' letters to patients in poor practices as Field unveils findings from first 1000 inspections. *Pulse*. 12 December.

Scrivens E (2007) The future of regulation and governance. *J R Soc Promot Health*. **127**(2): 72–7.

CHAPTER 4

Commissioning for quality improvement

SUMMARY

- Commissioning can drive improvements in the quality of healthcare.
- Stages of the commissioning cycle include assessing needs, setting priorities, contracting with providers and reviewing service delivery.
- Evidence from previous forms of primary care-led commissioning (PCLC) suggests that clinical commissioning groups (CCGs) may prove more effective at developing primary and intermediate care than shifting funds from hospital services.
- Successful commissioning requires managerial and financial expertise, accurate information and, crucially, the engagement of clinicians.

INTRODUCTION

The concept of healthcare commissioning has attracted widespread public and professional attention since the coalition government's reforming White Paper *Equity and Excellence: Liberating the NHS* was published in 2010 (Department of Health 2010). These proposals were revised and subsequently formalised in the Health and Social Care Act 2012, which focused on creating a clinician-led commissioning system that is sensitive to the needs of patients (Department of Health 2012).

In this chapter, we examine the nature of commissioning and its history, particularly in relation to commissioning as a driver for quality improvement. We then apply evidence relating to previous forms of PCLC to the establishment of CCGs. What does history suggest is needed for these new practice groupings to improve the quality of care through the processes of commissioning?

WHAT *IS* COMMISSIONING?

The term 'commissioning' emerged from the creation of a National Health Service (NHS) 'quasi-market' as part of the Conservative reforms of 1990 (Secretaries of State for Health 1989). Within this quasi-market ('quasi' because operations of this market were closely managed by government), the roles of planning and procuring (purchasing) care were formally separated from that of provision – the so-called purchaser–provider split.

It is the role of commissioners to secure, rather than directly provide, services that meet the needs of the populations for whose health they are responsible. There are four main steps involved in commissioning healthcare, often referred to as the commissioning 'cycle' (*see* Box 4.1), each of which provides opportunities for quality improvement.

BOX 4.1 Four stages of the commissioning cycle

1 Assessment of need
2 Setting priorities
3 Contracting with providers
4 Monitoring and reviewing service delivery

An assessment of need is essential to determine health inequalities and patients' unmet needs so that services can be targeted appropriately. Joint Strategic Needs Assessments help to identify local health needs, and commissioners need to identify inadequacies in service provision, cost, geographical distribution and quality when planning services and setting priorities.

Services may be designed or redesigned to meet the identified healthcare needs of the population, and contracting with providers is the process by which existing arrangements may be renegotiated, or new contracts drawn up that can directly affect the quality of care provided.

Monitoring and reviewing service delivery is the final stage of the cycle. Commissioners require accurate and timely information on the use and costs of services and quality of care, to assist them in making informed decisions about future commissioning arrangements, to ensure that they do not overspend and that quality is ensured.

Thus, commissioners are responsible for discriminating between providers to maximise value, seeking to influence providers in terms not just of price but also of service quality.

THE RISE OF 'PRIMARY CARE COMMISSIONING'

Since the 1990s, commissioning responsibilities have been divided between formal NHS agencies operating on behalf of large populations (often in the region of 200 000–500 000 people) and general practices acting alone or in groups. This latter form of commissioning (primary care-led) built on the role of the general practitioner (GP) as the 'gatekeeper' to hospital services. As the clinical decisions made by GPs (e.g. referrals, prescribing decisions) determine how resources are utilised, it was a natural step to align formal commissioning and budgetary responsibilities with those clinical responsibilities.

The 1990 reforms introduced GP fundholding as the first example of this type of PCLC. This initiative offered GPs financial incentives to reduce unnecessary utilisation of care, promote new community-based services, negotiate lower prices and improve quality – for example, through faster access to hospital treatment. GP fundholders were legally autonomous commissioners with real budgets for a limited range of services. Although there were modest successes with fundholding, most initiatives focused on small-scale new services, and many GPs lacked the skills and desire to take a population-based approach to planning (Goodwin 1998). Critics of fundholding argued that the system was unfair, generated inherent conflicts of interest, involved high transaction costs and fragmented the profession (Mays, *et al.* 2000).

Fundholding was abolished under the Labour government of 1997, and by 2002 primary care trusts (PCTs) had been introduced, which included the practices in a defined geographical area and averaged 170 000 people in size. Practice-based commissioning was an initiative launched in 2005 with the aim of improving GP engagement in the process, providing better resources for patients and using resources more effectively. It was designed to place commissioning powers in the hands of GPs, with 'notional' budgets held by the PCTs.

Recent analyses of practice-based commissioning initiatives have revealed that many GP commissioners focused on small-scale local pilots providing hospital services in community settings, and few took an interest in redesign of existing services or wider commissioning activities (Smith, *et al.* 2004). It was evident that practice-based commissioning seemed restricted to a small group of enthusiastic GPs in each PCT, and although there was widespread support for the initiative, this did not translate into active engagement. Conflicts of interest arose from the opportunity for GPs to be both providers and commissioners of their own service (thus subverting patient choice) and from the opportunity for PCTs to favour the services they themselves provided rather than tendering competitively for services commissioned under practice-based commissioning (Smith, *et al.* 2004).

THE FUTURE OF HEALTHCARE COMMISSIONING

Under the Health and Social Care Act 2012, power and responsibility for commissioning was devolved to GPs in CCGs in order to shift decision-making as close as possible to individual patients (Department of Health 2012). All general practices belong to a CCG, established as statutory bodies with responsibility for commissioning some £60 billion worth of healthcare services in 2014. Each CCG has an accountable officer and a chief financial officer, and each member practice shares accountability for delivering local commissioning decisions. For CCGs to function effectively, member practices need to agree shared objectives, membership criteria, a policy for information-sharing, a dispute resolution process and formalised practice responsibilities.

NHS England, previously the NHS Commissioning Board, is the interface between the government and healthcare spending. It has the role of setting and managing CCG budgets, providing clear national standards, supporting the development, and holding CCGs accountable for commissioning contracts. Certain specialist services, such as transplantation and tertiary cancer care, together with dentistry, pharmacy and general practice continue to be commissioned by the NHS England on a regional or national level. In addition, the NHS England Area Teams support CCGs by hosting clinical networks and senates, bringing together experts on certain diseases and service areas (such as cardiac and stroke care) to help inform their commissioning decisions.

CCGs have taken shape in the face of severe financial stringencies, tasked to help deliver the government's 4% efficiency target each year until 2015. Their particular challenge is to reduce the inexorable rise in emergency admissions and better meet the needs of frail older people with multiple conditions. The NHS Outcomes Framework incorporates targets relating to these aims.

WHAT IMPACT HAS COMMISSIONING HAD ON HEALTH SERVICES?

The different forms of PCLC discussed so far in this chapter have given rise to a canon of research literature, with sometimes inconsistent messages. The impact of PCLC in the past gives some indication of the likely impact of practice-based commissioning in the future (Smith and Mays 2012).

In their comprehensive review of the published evidence, Smith, *et al.* (2004) concluded starkly that 'there is little substantive research evidence to demonstrate that any commissioning approach has made a significant or strategic impact on secondary care services'. Given that the main policy objective of commissioning is to shape health systems around the needs of patients and, in particular, to shift funding from hospitals into the community, this is a disappointment.

It is outside the hospital domain that PCLC has proved most effective, with consistent evidence of the development of new services in primary and intermediate care, reductions in the costs of prescribing and new forms of quality assessment in primary care (Mays, *et al.* 2000).

However, PCLC also resulted in some negative outcomes that must be set against any benefits. That GP fundholding and total purchasing pilots resulted in service and quality inequities is generally accepted – and was inevitable, given that both schemes delivered benefits that were not universal. This was partly due to the tendency of fundholding to attract well-organised practices from better-off parts of the country, with inner-city practices particularly under-represented (Goodwin 1998).

REALISING THE BENEFITS OF PRIMARY CARE-LED COMMISSIONING

The evidence suggests that previous models of PCLC faced a number of common challenges that held back their development. These included organisational instability, clinical disengagement, insufficient management capacity and a lack of timely and accurate information on which to base their commissioning decisions (Smith, *et al.* 2006). The relatively modest impact of commissioners in the past might be significantly increased if support for PCLC is improved. What is required for CCGs to commission more successfully?

CLINICAL ENGAGEMENT

Perhaps the most fundamental impediment to PCLC is the limited involvement of clinicians. Direct involvement in decisions about resource allocation places the GP in the role of rationer, a task which many GPs feel uncomfortable with because it conflicts with their preferred role as their patient's advocate (Marshall and Harrison 2005). Moreover, patients may be less willing to accept the advice that they do need treatment or referral if they believe the GP's decision is influenced by budgetary considerations. Engendering collective responsibility among all practitioners for staying within budget or adhering to prescribing and referral protocols is difficult. The extent to which they will share a commitment to the needs of the locality as opposed to those of their own practice will crucially affect the development of PCLC.

VALID INFORMATION AND EVIDENCE

Much of the data used to assess health needs are based on electoral wards, i.e. geographical boundaries rather than practice boundaries. Practice boundaries do not necessarily fit into 'natural' communities, nor are they coterminous with local authority boundaries used by social services and other agencies. Coordination of information sources can be especially difficult in urban areas where practice selection effects operate more powerfully. Technical obstacles such as the difficulties of controlling for case mix are not easily resolved.

There appears to be no 'ideal' size for a commissioning organisation. Different population bases are needed for commissioning different services and there is little compelling evidence suggesting that bigger is necessarily better (Bojke, *et al.* 2001).

Just as evidence-based clinical practice applies the judicious use of the best evidence available when making decisions for individual patients, evidence-based commissioning implies the consistent use of evidence when planning populations' health services. The QIPP (Quality, Innovation, Productivity and Prevention) initiative models good practice but does not necessarily provide robust evidence on which to base purchasing decisions (National Institute for Health and Clinical Excellence 2012). NHS England is able to reward CCGs using quality premium payments to reflect the quality of services they commission and associated health outcomes.

MANAGERIAL EXPERTISE

Effective purchasing for quality in its widest sense requires a wide range of skills, including needs assessment, contracting, performance monitoring, accounting and budget management. Beyond an understanding of the processes of commissioning, some specialist knowledge is required to make strategically coherent purchasing decisions. CCGs require a range of skills such as the stratification of patients according to risk, advanced case management, predictive modelling of 'high user' patients, handling and analysis of routine data, and more refined assessment of service quality and outcomes (Smith, *et al.* 2006). These competencies are in short supply.

EQUITY AND PUBLIC HEALTH

It remains to be seen whether GPs and practice staff working in 'difficult' areas will have the time or the inclination to get involved in PCLC and whether the scheme will help to improve services in disadvantaged areas. CCGs in more deprived areas may struggle to defy the 'inverse care law', where poorer-quality services are associated with socio-economic deprivation whether at individual or population level (Tudor Hart 2000). CCGs include practices at different levels of development and quality. Practices with low inappropriate referral rates or efficient prescribing policies may be unwilling to share risk with practices perceived as less developed. On the other hand, closer working between more and less developed practices has most potential to raise the quality of primary care in a locality.

Preventive activities risk being ignored if PCLC focuses largely on secondary care. CCGs are represented on health and well-being boards, which provide strategic oversight of all areas of health and social care. In theory, practice-level budgets provide a motivating 'business case' for health promotion and disease prevention (Department of Health 2007). However, public health skills may be in short supply on CCGs. Health and well-being boards have yet to demonstrate their impact (O'Dowd 2013).

MEANINGFUL PUBLIC INVOLVEMENT

A commonly stated advantage of involving GPs in the commissioning process is that they are closer to patients and therefore can help to ensure that plans take account of patients' needs and preferences (Smith and Mays 2012). The assumption that the views and priorities of GPs are congruent with their patients' needs has not been tested. It will be important to monitor how CCGs make themselves accountable to the people on whose behalf they are securing services.

BOX 4.2 Case studies – 'Blue sky commissioning'

Some CCGs are seeking to improve their populations' health through closer links with local authorities (Kmietowicz 2014). In Bradford, for example, the three CCGs have invested £1.2 million in services to address hazardous drinking, which include assessment workers, a detox service and community intensive support teams and an Eastern European service. In Leicester, two CCGs are investing £1.5 million in services to support troubled families, while NHS Oldham CCG is contributing to a warm homes scheme. These kinds of innovative, 'up-stream' investments in public health beyond the NHS have the potential to save money but can nevertheless be hard to defend when the benefits accrue to other budgets and only in the longer term.

CONCLUSION

These developments represent a continuing evolution of previous commissioning initiatives but CCGs exist in a different world to those of their predecessors. Since 2010 the government has introduced further market-oriented reforms designed to intensify competition among providers, embrace the private sector and provide more rights for patients to choose where they receive treatment.

The focus of commissioning is now on the creation and shaping of markets as much as on the allocation of resources directly to providers. Opponents of these reforms warn of wholesale privatisation within the NHS; markets may drive down costs but may drive down quality also. The government's regulations on competition in the NHS remain ambiguous (McKee 2013).

CCGs exercise some influence over their constituent practices but have limited responsibilities for the commissioning of primary care. Levelling up the quality of services provided at the front line would surely be their greatest legacy in terms of population health.

BOX 4.3 Factors likely to increase the effectiveness of commissioning

- Strong, skilled leadership
- Organisational stability
- A blend of incentives, financial and non-financial, to promote clinical engagement
- Access to high-quality, up-to-date information at practice level to evaluate and inform commissioning decisions
- Worthwhile in-service training opportunities for those leading CCGs
- Even distribution of the managerial resources required to underpin commissioning
- Tried and tested mechanisms of public accountability

The past is not always a faithful guide to the future but previous experience is illuminating (Curry, *et al.* 2008). The new NHS environment may, in certain respects, be more conducive to effective commissioning but the historical limitations to PCLC are likely to recur. Many challenges will need to be overcome if CCGs are to survive for longer than their predecessors and contribute effectively to the quality agenda.

REFERENCES

Bojke C, Gravelle H, Wilkin D (2001) Is bigger better for primary care groups and trusts? *BMJ.* **322**(7286): 599–602.

Curry N, Goodwin N, Naylor C, *et al.* (2008) *Practice-based commissioning: reinvigorate, replace or abandon?* The King's Fund: London.

Department of Health (2012) *Health and Social Care Act.* Department of Health: London.

Department of Health (2010) *Equity and excellence: liberating the NHS.* The Stationery Office: Norwich.

Department of Health (2007) *Commissioning framework for health and well-being.* Department of Health: London.

Goodwin N (1998) GP fundholding. In: Le Grand J, Mays N, Mulligan J (eds). *Learning from the NHS internal market.* The King's Fund: London.

Kmietowicz Z (2014) Blue sky commissioning. *BMJ.* **348**: g285.

Marshall M, Harrison S (2005) It's about more than money: financial incentives and internal motivation. *Qual Saf Health Care.* **14**(1): 4–5.

Mays N, Mulligan JA, Goodwin N (2000) The British quasi-market in health care: a balance sheet of the evidence. *J Health Serv Res Policy.* **5**(1): 49–58.

McKee M (2013) The future of England's health care lies in the hands of competition lawyers. *BMJ.* **346**: f1733.

National Institute for Health and Clinical Excellence (2012) *Process manual for the Quality and Productivity programme: a guide for stakeholders.* NICE: London.

O'Dowd A (2013) Some health and wellbeing boards are too 'pink and fluffy' and lack spine, expert warns. *BMJ.* **346**: f136.

Secretaries of State for Health (1989) *Working for patients.* CM 555. HMSO: London.

Smith JA, Lewis R, Harrison T (2006) *Making commissioning effective in the reformed NHS in England.* Health Policy Forum: London.

Smith JA, Mays N (2012) GP led commissioning: time for a cool appraisal. *BMJ.* **344**: e980.

Smith JA, Mays N, Dixon J, *et al.* (2004) *A review of the effectiveness of primary care-led commissioning and its place in the UK NHS.* The Health Foundation: London.

Tudor Hart J (2000) Commentary: three decades of the inverse care law. *BMJ.* **320**(7226): 18–19.

.

SECTION 2

Tools for improvement

CHAPTER 5

Frameworks for improvement

SUMMARY

- Quality is about increasing desired health outcomes; patients may have different views from healthcare professionals on the outcomes desired.
- Commonly used frameworks for improvement include clinical audit, the plan-do-study-act (PDSA) cycle and significant event analysis (SEA).
- All three techniques involve systematic analysis of current practice, reflection on what we are trying to achieve and – crucially – action to effect change.
- Closely related to SEA, root cause analysis (RCA) tries to identify the underlying causes of problems, as opposed to simply addressing their symptoms.
- Thorough record keeping, acknowledgement of the need to change and negotiation across the team are necessary for improvement to result.

INTRODUCTION

Quality has been defined as:

> the degree to which health services for individuals and populations increase the likelihood of desired health outcomes and are consistent with current professional knowledge. (Gray 1997)

Outcomes can be viewed from different stakeholder's perspectives. The 'desired' outcomes may be subtly different for managers, patients and clinicians.

Patients clearly want treatment that works and place a high priority on how that treatment is delivered. Clinicians focus on effectiveness and want to provide treatment that works best for each of their patients. Managers are rightly concerned with efficiency and seek to maximise the population health gain through best use of increasingly limited budgets. The range of different outcomes desired demonstrates the multidimensional nature of quality. The first stage in any attempt to measure quality is therefore to think about what dimensions are important for you.

EVALUATING QUALITY

Evaluation (considered in more detail in Chapter 10) has been defined as:

> a process that attempts to determine, as systematically and objectively as possible the relevance, effectiveness and impact of activities in the light of their objectives, e.g. evaluation of structure, process and outcome, clinical trials, quality of care (Last 1995).

Where do we start when thinking about evaluation of a service in the National Health Service? Avedis Donabedian (1966) distinguished four elements:

1 Structure (buildings, staff, equipment)
2 Process (all that is done to patients)
3 Outputs (immediate results of medical intervention)
4 Outcomes (gains in health status).

Thus, for example, evaluation of new screening algorithms for early detection of cancer in primary care (Hippisley-Cox and Coupland 2013b; Hippisley-Cox and Coupland 2013a) will need to consider:

- the cost of implementing the programme (additional consultations, investigations and referrals)
- the numbers of patients screened, coverage rates for defined age ranges and sex, number and proportion of patients screened who are referred, time to referral from first consultation or number of consultations before referral (process)
- number of new cancers identified, numbers of true and false positives and negatives treatments performed (outputs)
- cancer incidence, prevalence and mortality rates together with patient experience (outcomes).

This distinction is helpful because for many interventions it may be difficult to obtain robust data on health outcomes unless large numbers are scrutinised over long periods. For example, when evaluating the quality of hypertension management within a general practice, you may be reliant on intermediate outcome or process measures (the proportion of the appropriate population screened, treated and adequately controlled) as a proxy for health status outcomes.

The assumption here is that evidence from larger-scale studies showing that control of hypertension reduces subsequent death rates from heart disease will be reflected in your own practice population's health experience. There are three main types of quality measure in healthcare: (1) consumer ratings, (2) clinical performance data and (3) effects on individual and population health (*see* Chapter 7).

THE MODEL FOR IMPROVEMENT

The Institute for Healthcare Improvement's (www.ihi.org) model for improvement provides the basis for the commonly used quality improvement techniques of clinical audit and PDSA cycles (Institute for Healthcare Improvement 2013; Plsek 1999). It is summarised in three simple questions:

1 What are we trying to achieve?

2   How will we know if we have improved?
3   What changes can we make to improve?

How these questions are applied in practical frameworks for improvement is described in more detail shortly.

CLINICAL AUDIT

The clinical audit cycle (*see* Figure 5.1) involves measuring performance and implementing change against one or more predefined criteria against a standard until that standard is achieved or until a new standard is set. Clinical audit can be effective in improving processes and outcomes of care (Holden 2004; Jamtvedt, *et al.* 2003) but this is often hindered by inadequate methods (Hearnshaw, *et al.* 2003; Bowie, *et al.* 2007). The greatest challenge is to make necessary adjustments and re-evaluate performance – in other words, to complete the cycle.

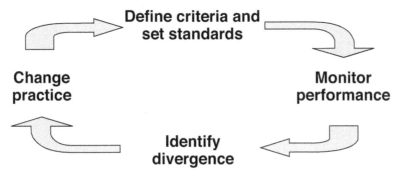

FIGURE 5.1 The clinical audit cycle

Clinical audit is therefore a systematic process involving the following stages.
- **Identify the problem or issue.** Selecting an audit topic should answer the question, 'What needs to be improved and why?' This is likely to reflect national or local standards and guidelines where there is definitive evidence about effective clinical practice. The topic should focus on areas where problems have been encountered in practice.
- **Define criteria and standards.** Audit criteria are explicit statements that define what elements of care are being measured (e.g. 'patients with asthma should have a care plan.'). The standard defines the level of care to be achieved for each criterion (e.g. 'care plans have been agreed for over 80% of patients with asthma'). Standards are usually agreed by consensus but may also be based on published evidence (e.g. childhood vaccination rates that confer population herd immunity) or on the results of a previous (local, national or published) audit.
- **Monitor performance.** To ensure that only essential information is collected, details of what is to be measured must be established from the outset. Sample sizes for data collection are often a compromise between the statistical validity of the results and the resources available for data collection and analysis.
- **Compare performance with criteria and standards.** This stage identifies

divergences between actual results and standards sets. Were the standards met and if not, why not?

- **Implement change.** Once the results of the audit have been discussed, an agreement must be reached about recommendations for change. Using an action plan to record these recommendations is good practice. This should include who has agreed to do what and by when. Each point needs to be well defined, with an individual named as responsible for it, and an agreed timescale for its completion.
- **Complete the cycle to sustain improvements.** After an agreed period, the audit should be repeated. The same strategies for identifying the sample, methods and data analysis should be used to ensure comparability with the original audit. The re-audit should demonstrate that any changes have been implemented and improvements have been made. Further changes may then be required, leading to additional re-audits. An example audit is shown in Box 5.1.

BOX 5.1 Audit record example

Title of the audit: Audit of management of obese patients

Reason for the choice of topic: All team members have noted the increasing prevalence of overweight and obesity across the practice population.

Dates of the first data collection and the re-audit: 1 March 2013 and 1 September 2013

Criteria to be audited and the standards set:
- *Criterion* – the health records of adults with a BMI>30 should contain a multi-component weight management plan.
- *Standard* – 100%. According to National Institute for Health and Care Excellence guidelines, adult patients with a BMI>30 should have a documented multi-component weight management plan setting out strategies for addressing changes in diet and activity levels, developed with the relevant healthcare professional. The plan should be explicit about the targets for each of the components for the individual patient and the specific strategies for that patient. A copy of the plan should be retained in the health record and monitored by the relevant healthcare professional.

Results of the first data collection: Of 72 patients with documented BMI>30, only 8 (11%) had copies of weight management plans in their records.

Summary of the discussion and changes agreed: The results were reviewed at the next clinical governance meeting, where it was felt that hard copies for the paper record were less important than documentation of the process in the electronic record.

Results of the second data collection: Of 48 patients with BMI>30, 16 (33%) had documented weight management plans in their electronic record.

Point to ponder
- Can you think of an audit you would like to undertake? Why is it needed? What criteria and standards would you set?

THE PLAN-DO-STUDY-ACT CYCLE

The PDSA cycle takes audit one stage further (*see* Figure 5.2) by focusing on the development, testing and implementation of quality improvement (Institute for Healthcare Improvement 2013; Plsek 1999).

The PDSA cycle involves repeated, rapid, small-scale tests of change, carried out in sequence (i.e. changes tested one after another) or in parallel (different people or groups testing different changes), to see whether and to what extent the changes work, before implementing one or more of these changes on a larger scale. The following stages are involved: first, develop a plan and define the objective (plan); second, carry out the plan and collect data (do); third, analyse the data and summarise what was learned (study); fourth, implement any changes required before going on to plan the next cycle with necessary modifications (act).

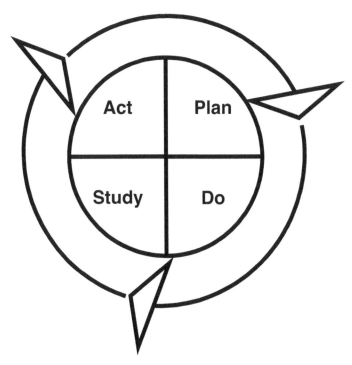

FIGURE 5.2 The plan-do-study-act cycle

- **Plan.** Develop a plan for the change(s) to be tested or implemented. Make predictions about what will happen and why. Develop a plan to test the change. (Who? What? When? Where? What data need to be collected?)

- **Do.** Carry out the test by implementing the change.
- **Study.** Look at data before and after the change. Usually this involves using run or control charts together with qualitative feedback. Compare the data to your predictions. Reflect on what was learned and summarise this.
- **Act.** Plan the next test, determining what modifications should be made. Prepare a plan for the next test. Decide to fully implement one or more successful changes. An example is shown in Box 5.2 and associated Figures 5.3 and 5.4.

BOX 5.2 Example of a quality improvement project

Title: Improving monitoring of azathioprine

Date completed: 1 June 2012

Description: This was a quality improvement project focusing on improving monitoring of commonly used disease-modifying antirheumatic (immunosuppressant) drugs (DMARDs, i.e. methotrexate, azathioprine) in the practice.

Reason for the choice of topic and statement of the problem: DMARDs are commonly prescribed under shared care arrangements with specialists. The general practitioner has a responsibility for ensuring that the drugs are appropriately monitored for evidence of bone marrow suppression and liver dysfunction.

Priorities for improvement and the measurements adopted: The aim of this quality improvement project was to improve monitoring of the two most commonly used DMARDs in the practice, methotrexate and azathioprine. The criteria agreed for monitoring were:
- methotrexate – full blood count and liver function tests performed within the previous 3 months
- azathioprine – full blood count performed within the previous 3 months; renal function within the past 6 months.

Baseline data collection and analysis: The first data collection presented in the run and control charts from week 1 to 6 showed inadequate blood monitoring of these drugs with rates of complete blood monitoring for 10 patients (four patients prescribed methotrexate and six prescribed azathioprine) on these drugs at around 70% (*see* Figures 5.3 and 5.4).

Quality improvement: The team met to plan how to measure monitoring and how to improve this. Clinical and administrative staff discussed the topic. During the baseline measurements for 6 weeks, improvements were planned. The first improvement introduced was a protocol for a search and prescription reminder for patients on these drugs. All patients receiving DMARDs were put on a 3-month prescription recall and an automatic prescription reminder to attend for blood monitoring at every 3-month recall was set up. Following an initial improvement to 80% compliance with monitoring it

---

was decided to send a written recall letter for blood tests and a follow-up appointment with the doctor.

The results of the second data collection: The subsequent data collection showed monitoring rates consistently at 100%.

Intervention and the maintenance of successful changes: We provided a system for more consistent monitoring of DMARDs.

Quality improvement achieved and reflections on the process: This project enabled members of the practice to improve their knowledge in this area. This led to higher-quality, safer care for patients.

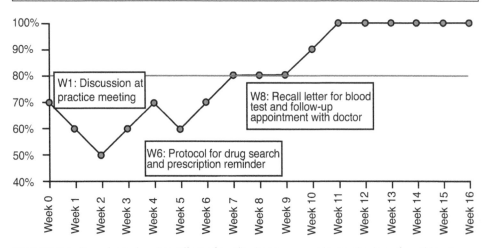

FIGURE 5.3 Run chart showing effect of quality improvement in monitoring of azathioprine

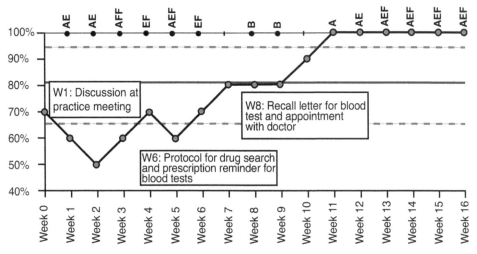

FIGURE 5.4 Control chart showing effect of quality improvement in monitoring of azathioprine (W1 = week one; W6 = week six; W8 = week 8)

SIGNIFICANT EVENT ANALYSIS

SEA is a very different approach to quality improvement, involving the structured investigation of individual episodes that have been identified by a member or members of the healthcare team as 'significant' (*see* Box 5.3). SEA improves the quality and safety of patient care by encouraging reflective learning and, where necessary, the implementation of change to minimise recurrence of adverse events or increase likelihood of positive events in question (Pringle 2000). It can improve risk management, it can enhance patient safety and it facilitates the reporting of patient safety incidents by healthcare practitioners.

SEA has been described as the process by which

> individual cases, in which there has been a significant occurrence (not necessarily involving an undesirable outcome for the patient), are analysed in a systematic and detailed way to ascertain what can be learned about the overall quality of care and to indicate changes that might lead to future improvements. (National Patient Safety Agency 2013)

The aim of SEA is to:
- gather and map information to determine what happened
- identify problems with healthcare delivery
- identify contributory factors and root causes
- agree what needs to change and implement solutions.

BOX 5.3 Common types of significant events

- Prescribing error
- Failure to action an abnormal result
- Failure to diagnose
- Failure to refer
- Failure to deal with an emergency call
- Breach in confidentiality
- Breakdown in communication

COMMON CAUSES OF SIGNIFICANT EVENTS

There are many types of significant event. Most are multifactorial in origin, and for this reason SEA often explores issues such as the following.
- **Information:** for example, potentially important data overlooked on co-morbidities (e.g. previous bronchospasm when considering beta blockers), previous drug side effects, allergies or potential interactions.
- **Patient factors:** for example, the doctor failed to check that the patient understood the reasons for treatment, the dosing, timing and the stop and start dates, and failed to check that the patient knew the possible side effects.
- **Professional factors:** poor communication skills; lack of medical knowledge or skills; mistakes due to pressure of time, unnecessary interruptions, stress, and so forth.

- **Systems failure:** for example, lack of education, training or supervision; poor identification of roles and responsibilities; lack of detailed guidelines, protocols, and so forth; lack of audit or regular reviews.

SIX STEPS IN SIGNIFICANT EVENT ANALYSIS

1 **Identify and record** significant events for analysis and highlight these at a suitable meeting. Enable staff to routinely record significant events using a logbook or pro forma.
2 **Collect factual information** including written and electronic records, the thoughts and opinions of those involved in the event. This may include patients or relatives or healthcare professionals based outside the practice.
3 **Meet to discuss and analyse** the event(s) with all relevant members of the team. The meeting should be conducted in an open, fair, honest and non-threatening atmosphere. Notes of the meeting should be taken and circulated. Meetings should be held routinely, perhaps as part of monthly team meetings, when all events of interest can be discussed and analysed allowing all relevant staff to offer their thoughts and suggestions. The person you choose to facilitate a significant event meeting or to take responsibility for an event analysis again will depend on team dynamics and staff confidence.
4 Undertake a structured analysis of the event. The focus should be on establishing exactly what happened and why. The main emphasis is on learning from the event and changing behaviours, practices or systems, where appropriate. The purpose of the analysis is to minimise the chances of an event recurring. (On rare occasions it may not be possible to implement change – for example, the likelihood of the event happening again may be very small, or change may be out of your control. If so, clearly document why you have not taken action.)
5 **Monitor the progress** of actions that are agreed and implemented by the team. For example, if the head receptionist agrees to design and introduce a new protocol for taking telephone messages, then progress on this new development should be reported back at a future meeting.
6 **Write up the SEA** once changes have been agreed. This provides documentary evidence that the event has been dealt with. It is good practice to attach any additional evidence (e.g. a copy of a letter or an amended protocol) to the report.

The report should be written up by the individual who led on the event analysis and should include the following:
- date of event
- date of meeting
- lead investigator
- what happened?
- why did it happen?
- what has been learned?
- what has been changed?

It is good practice to keep the report anonymous so that individuals and other organisations cannot be identified.

Purists may wish to seek educational feedback on the SEA once it has been written up. Research has repeatedly shown that around one-third of event analyses are unsatisfactory, mainly because the team has failed to understand why the event happened or to take necessary action to prevent recurrence (McKay, *et al.* 2009). Sharing the SEA with others, such as a group of general practitioners or practice managers, provides an opportunity for them to comment on your event analysis and also learn from what you have done.

BOX 5.4 Significant event analysis record

Date of report: 12 March 2014

Reporter: AB

Patient identifier: 1234

Date of event: 15 February 2014

Summary of event:
While entering data on her template, Nurse X noticed a previous glucose of 7.7 recorded on 3 February 2014. She initially assumed that this was normal because the template did not distinguish between fasting and random glucose tests. She checked the result and found that it was in fact a fasting glucose, which may have indicated diabetes. Nurse X explained the problem to the patient, apologised and checked whether she had any symptoms or complications. The patient was adhering to her diet and was asymptomatic. Nurse X arranged for a repeat fasting glucose, cholesterol, thyroid function, electrolytes and HbA1c and to review the patient with the results of these investigations. The fasting glucose came back as 8.8 mmol/L (normal less than 6.0 mmol/L), confirming diabetes.

Discussion points:
The template was unclear and made this error more likely

Agreed action points:
Adjust template to distinguish between fasting and random glucose.

Responsible person:
AB

Point to ponder
- Can you think of an SEA you have been involved with? What happened? What action was undertaken? What would have increased its impact?

Closely related to SEA, root cause analysis (RCA) is a method of problem-solving that tries to identify the underlying causes of problems, as opposed to simply addressing their symptoms (National Patient Safety Agency 2013). Like clinical audit and PDSA, RCA and SEA are closely interlinked. By focusing correction on root causes, problem recurrence can be prevented. RCA is typically used as a reactive method of identifying event(s) causes, revealing problems and solving them. Analysis is done *after* an event has occurred. Insights derived from RCA may also be used proactively to predict probable events even *before* they occur. RCA is not a single, sharply defined methodology; many different tools, processes, and philosophies are used in performing RCA.

TABLE 5.1 Comparing clinical audit, plan-do-study-act (PDSA) and significant event analysis (SEA)

	Clinical audit	PDSA	SEA
Example triggers	Significant event, previous audit, clinical guideline	Significant event, previous audit, clinical guideline	Significant event (critical incident, complaint, success)
Review of evidence for change	Yes	Yes	Sometimes
Criteria	Yes	Yes	No
Standards	Yes	No	No
Type of measurement	Before and after	Continuous (statistical process control)	No: detailed review of a single event
Change implementation strategy	Change(s) implemented together after first audit	Often multiple changes conducted in sequence or parallel	Recommendation for change in policy, protocol, structure or behaviour
Cyclical	Yes	Yes	No
Ideal outcome	To meet or exceed standard	To improve from baseline	Analysis leading to change in process

CONCLUSION

Clinical audit, PDSA and SEA are compared in Table 5.1. All three techniques involve gaining a deeper understanding and reflecting on what we are trying to achieve and what changes can be made to improve. SEA is now routinely used in UK general practice as part of the requirement for revalidation of doctors. Clinical audit is also commonly used, although many 'audits' do not complete the cycle. PDSA cycles are less well understood by many practitioners and most have little practical experience of PDSA. Clinical audit and PDSA use a measurement process before and after implementing one or more changes to assess whether improvement has actually occurred. However, in clinical audit this is usually a single measure before and after the change, whereas PDSA involves continuous repeated measurement using statistical process control with run or control charts (*see* Figures 7.1 and 7.3, respectively; *see* Chapter 7). SEA should ideally lead to changes in policy or practice but does not involve measuring the effects of this. The main difference between clinical audit and PDSA is that audit involves implementation of change after the first measurement followed by a further measurement, whereas PDSA involves continuous measurement during implementation of multiple changes conducted in sequence (i.e. one after the other) or in parallel (i.e. different individuals or groups implementing different changes at the same time).

FURTHER READING

- Berwick DM (1996) A primer on leading the improvement of systems. *BMJ.* **312**(7031): 619–22.
- Pringle M, Royal College of General Practitioners (1995) *Significant event auditing: a study of the feasibility and potential of case-based auditing in primary medical care.* Royal College of General Practitioners: London.

REFERENCES

Bowie P, Cooke S, Lo P, *et al.* (2007) The assessment of criterion audit cycles by external peer review: when is an audit not an audit? *J Eval Clin Pract.* **13**(3): 352–7.

Donabedian A (1966) Evaluating the quality of medical care. *Milbank Mem Fund Q.* 44(3 Suppl.): 166–206.

Gray JAM (1997) *Evidence-based healthcare: how to make health policy and management decisions.* Churchill Livingstone: New York, NY.

Hearnshaw HM, Harker RM, Cheater FM, *et al.* (2003) Are audits wasting resources by measuring the wrong things? A survey of methods used to select audit review criteria. *Qual Saf Health Care.* **12**(1): 24–8.

Hippisley-Cox J, Coupland C (2013a) Symptoms and risk factors to identify men with suspected cancer in primary care: derivation and validation of an algorithm. *Br J Gen Pract.* **63**(606): e1–10.

Hippisley-Cox J, Coupland C (2013b) Symptoms and risk factors to identify women with suspected cancer in primary care: derivation and validation of an algorithm. *Br J Gen Pract.* **63**(606): e11–21.

Holden JD (2004) Systematic review of published multi-practice audits from British general practice. *J Eval Clin Pract.* **10**(2): 247–72.

Institute for Healthcare Improvement (2013) *Science of improvement: testing changes.* Institute for Healthcare Improvement: Cambridge, MA.

Jamtvedt G, Young JM, Kristoffersen DT, *et al.* (2003) Audit and feedback: effects on professional practice and health care outcomes. *Cochrane Database Syst Rev.* (3): CD000259.

Last JM (1995). *A dictionary of epidemiology third edition.* International Epidemiological Association. Oxford University Press: Oxford.

McKay J, Bradley N, Lough M, *et al.* (2009). A review of significant events analysed in general practice: implications for the quality and safety of patient care. *BMC Fam.* **10**: 61.

National Patient Safety Agency (2013) *Root Cause Analysis (RCA) tools: getting started.* Department of Health: London.

Plsek PE (1999) Quality improvement methods in clinical medicine. *Pediatrics.* **103**(1 Suppl. E): 203–14.

Pringle M (2000) Significant event auditing. *Scand J Prim Health Care.* **18**: 200–2.

CHAPTER 6

Understanding processes and how to improve them

SUMMARY

- Understanding healthcare processes is vital in order to improve them.
- Logic models help to determine what information to collect to understand processes and how to analyse this information to design more reliable and higher-quality healthcare processes.
- Data on processes can be collected using surveys, interviews or direct observations.
- Processes can be analysed using process maps, critical-to-quality trees, driver diagrams and cause and effect diagrams.

INTRODUCTION

Many quality improvement methods in healthcare are directed at improving processes. This can be achieved by understanding processes, by mapping the steps involved and analysing these, to eliminate wasteful steps and reinforce steps that deliver better care. The aim is to reduce unintended variation, increase reliability of the process and deliver high-quality care consistently.

To some, the idea of 'process' may sound overly mechanistic; it may resemble the notion of industrial processes in manufacturing and the conveyor belt or a factory line. Linked to this is the implication that reliability and consistency means treating everyone the same, whatever their needs. These are basic misconceptions: a misunderstanding of what is meant by 'process' and by 'reliability'.

If we look more deeply into these ideas we see that the underlying principles are the same whether for manufacturing or service industries, including health, an idea that W Edwards Deming understood and explained over half a century ago (Deming 1982). As we examine the idea of processes and reliability, we will draw on work from the intellectual giants of the quality improvement movement including Deming (1982), Joseph Juran (Juran and Godfrey 1999) and more recently Davis Balestracci (2009).

There are some basic assumptions here that need to be clarified: quality healthcare is that which is effective, safe and improves patient experience (Darzi of Denham 2008). Processes can be defined as a series of activities or inputs that lead to outputs: inputs include people, work methods, equipment, materials, measurements and environment. Understanding and improving processes can reduce inappropriate and unintended variation. In this chapter we examine these ideas in turn.

PROCESSES

All work is a process (Balestracci 2009). Healthcare processes are the steps that are taken or involve, either explicitly or implicitly, whether sequentially or in parallel, by people or machines, carrying out activities that are designed to improve or maintain health. For example, the process of a referral to hospital can involve the decision to refer (a cognitive process), following discussion with a patient of his or her needs or wants, a communication (e.g. letter) transferred to the hospital, and an electronic appointment, letter or telephone call to the patient to let him or her know a date or time of an appointment.

This example is relatively straightforward compared with many health processes, which are often more complex. Health processes may involve many more steps, actors, equipment, materials, environments and interactions between these. The timing of an appointment (one possible output measure) can vary depending on how this is measured, as well as other inputs such as the content of the referral letter, the material used (paper versus electronic), how it is sent (post versus electronic) and all of this can affect patient experience of the referral. A delayed or lost referral can lead to a poor patient experience, waste (the patient calling the surgery to find out when the referral will be), rework (resending the referral), additional costs and poor outcomes including premature death (e.g. for a patient with cancer who has a referral delayed).

A better understanding and fine-tuning of processes can make them more reliable and reduce inappropriate or unintended variation. In relation to health, this can improve effectiveness, safety and people's experience of healthcare. Quality healthcare meets patients' needs by improving their health, increasing levels of satisfaction and reducing errors (Juran and Godfrey 1999). To understand how to improve care, we need to understand how to improve the processes involved, to understand how to reduce inappropriate or unintended variation in these processes, and to understand how to make processes more consistent and reliable where this is required to improve outcomes of care. An important rider to applying these concepts in health systems is that some variation is inherent in the different presentations of disease, differences between patients and differences in choices of individuals (Starfield and Mangin 2010).

A number of conceptual and practical tools are available for understanding and improving processes and we will examine some of these. The range of tools considered in this chapter is not comprehensive but includes those we consider the most important and practically useful (*see* Box 6.1).

Point to ponder
- Consider which processes you would like to focus on to improve your practice.

ANALYTICAL TOOLS

A useful starting point for understanding and improving processes is the *logic model* (*see* Figure 6.1). The logic model defines what exactly we are trying to improve (the aims or priorities for improvement), describes who we are trying to improve it for (the population for which improvement is intended) and explains why we are trying to improve a particularly area of healthcare (the problem identified as in need of improvement). The model next describes the inputs, which include people, work methods, equipment, materials, environment and measurements. It also describes how we will go about improving care in terms of who we will involve (the participants), what they will do to bring about improvement (the activities) and what we wish to achieve in terms of processes (the outputs) that are intended, or have been shown, to lead to longer-term benefits. Benefits are described in terms of health or wider gains as well as possible harms (the outcomes), whether intended or incidental and in the short, medium or longer term (Medeiros, *et al.* 2005).

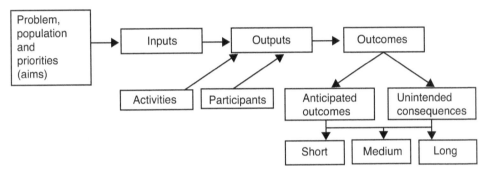

FIGURE 6.1 Logic model for analysing and improving processes

> **Point to ponder**
> ● Construct a logic model for a process you would like to improve (*see* Figure 6.4).

Various activities can help us understand the elements involved, and this understanding can then be used to improve them (*see* Box 6.1). For example, the problem, population of interest and priorities for improvement can be elucidated using interviews or surveys of patients and staff or direct observation.

Patients' views of what is important to them, how to meet their needs for better health, improve their experience, and reduce harms can be discerned by asking them directly about these issues. We can do this through the use of *interviews* or *focus groups*, *surveys* or *direct observation* of patients in their interactions with the health system (*see* Chapter 1). Patients may also share written accounts or audio/video diaries (Kyle, *et al.* 2011).

> **Points to ponder**
> ● How do you gather patients' views of what is important to them?
> ● How might you do this better?

Often, it can be helpful to ask practitioners the same question – that is, what constitutes good care and how can care be improved? Sometimes patients and practitioners agree but at other times their views may be discrepant. For example, patients' and practitioners' views on how to improve care of insomnia (Dyas, *et al.* 2010) or acute pain (Iqbal, *et al.* 2012), although broadly concordant, differ in some significant areas.

A *process map* is a tool to show pictorially the series of steps in a process of care or a patient journey. This can be constructed very simply by writing down the steps of a process on 'post-it' notes and connecting these on a large piece of paper using arrows. This is best done with the team or group involved in the process and concerned with improving it. Constructing the process map leads naturally to analysing it.

Often this exercise reveals a great many steps and complex interconnections between them, some of which are redundant, are unhelpful, are duplications or waste time and resources. Process maps are sometimes called 'spaghetti diagrams' to convey the intricate linkages between many steps. These processes can be confusing, conflicting, complex, chaotic and costly – Balestracci (2009) refers to these as the 'five Cs'.

The process map as well as showing redundant or wasteful steps can also help us to identify which steps in a process are critical to quality. This enables unhelpful or harmful steps to be removed. These measurable characteristics of a process, where standards need to be achieved to meet the quality requirements of the user, can be summarised using a *critical-to-quality tree*.

BOX 6.1 Activities for understanding and improving processes

Problem, population and priorities
- Interviews (discovery, narrative), focus groups
- Patient or practitioner surveys
- Direct observation

Inputs
- Process maps
- Cause and effect ('fishbone') diagram
- Driver diagrams
- Critical-to-quality trees

Outputs
- Process or outcome indicators/measures

The inputs can be expanded, either as a whole or in specific areas to form a *'cause and effect'* (*sometimes call a fishbone or Ishikawa*) *diagram* (*see* Figure 6.2). The diagram helps elucidate the causes of a problem and is an aid to finding solutions. The central line represents the patient pathway leading to the outcome of interest and this is affected by various inputs, including patients themselves (Medeiros, *et al.* 2005). The inputs include people, both patients and healthcare staff; work methods and organisational processes; equipment such as machines and materials; and the environment, which incorporates features such as policies, guidelines, protocols and organisational culture. Each in turn is influenced by various factors (represented by the subsidiary arrows).

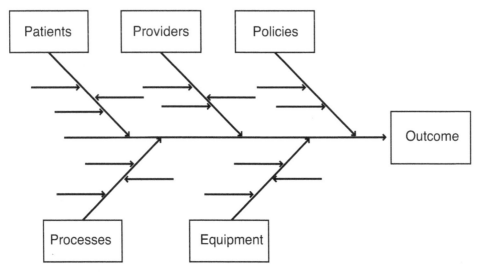

FIGURE 6.2 Cause and effect ('fishbone') diagram

Processes can also be summarised using a *driver diagram*. Driver diagrams enable a high-level improvement goal to be translated into a logical set of underpinning goals ('primary drivers') and specific actions ('secondary drivers') that can also be converted to measures. There are three stages to improving reliability (Nolan, *et al.* 2013), as represented in a driver diagram in Figure 6.3.

The first stage involves preventing failure, which can be achieved through standardisation of processes using guidelines and protocols, checklists for practitioners, feedback to individual staff or groups, and education and training for staff. The next stage involves provider prompts and 'forcing functions', which prevent failure by ensuring that a (critical-to-quality) process is completed before another can be undertaken. The final phase involves further redesign of the system to ensure that the process is as 'lean' as possible, minimising wasteful steps, reducing rework, reducing the chances of failure and maximising the efficient delivery of the process (*see* Figure 6.3).

Point to ponder
- How might you redesign a healthcare process in your practice using the tools described?

An example of this approach is shown for improving influenza vaccination rates in at-risk groups in primary care using a logic model (*see* Figure 6.4) and case study (*see* Box 6.2).

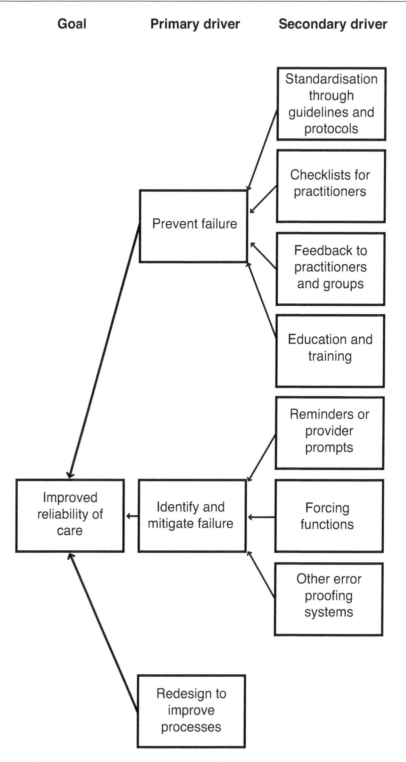

FIGURE 6.3 Driver diagram to improve reliability of care

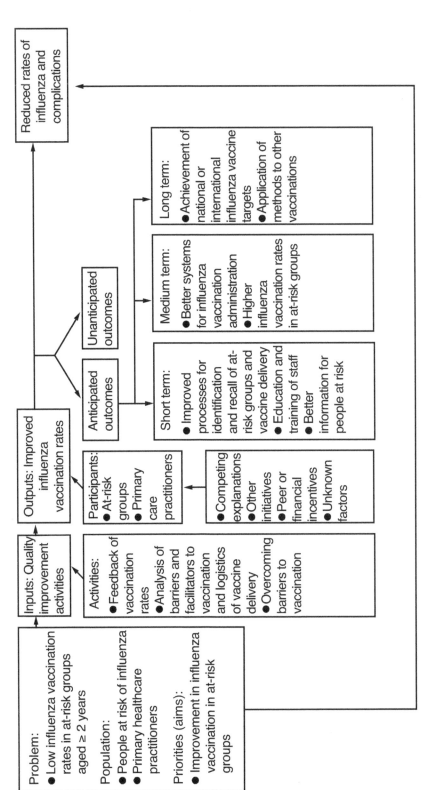

FIGURE 6.4 Improving influenza vaccination rates: logic model

BOX 6.2 Case study – improving influenza vaccination

Background: problem, population and priorities

Influenza (flu) is a common, potentially severe, but preventable infection that places a high burden on patients and healthcare providers. A safe, effective vaccine is offered annually by general practices to at-risk groups in the United Kingdom. People in high-risk groups including older people aged 65 years or over and those aged 2 years or over with specific conditions (heart disease, lung disease, diabetes, chronic kidney, liver or neurological disease and immunosuppression) make up 27% of the population and have a higher chance of severe influenza infection or its complications. There are 36 deaths per 100 000 of the population in the United Kingdom (an additional 12 000 per year) due directly to influenza, and of these, approximately two-thirds are in a vaccination risk group, whereas only a quarter receive vaccination. Uptake of seasonal influenza vaccination in the United Kingdom's at-risk population is below the national and international target of 75%. The number of influenza vaccinations needed to prevent one death is 120. We aimed to improved influenza vaccination rates in at-risk groups in primary care.

Identifying strategies: activities

We elucidated key strategies that were associated with higher rates of influenza vaccination through reviewing the research and surveying patients and practitioners. These included patient factors such as perception of being at-risk of influenza, a belief in vaccine effectiveness and fewer concerns about vaccine side effects; provider factors such as clear guidelines, consistent advice from the primary care team, and vaccination reminders and information for those patients in high-risk groups eligible for influenza vaccination; organisational factors such as identifying a lead member of staff responsible for running the vaccination campaign, identifying a lead member of staff to identify eligible patients, using the practice computer system to identify eligible patients more accurately, sending personal invitations to all eligible patients, working with community nurses and midwives to offer/provide vaccination to housebound and pregnant women, respectively, continuing vaccination until targets are achieved, and reviewing the success and actions of those involved in the influenza campaign (Dexter, *et al.* 2012).

Implementing changes: inputs

We used a combination of strategies for improving influenza vaccination rates including guidelines, practice leaflet and poster campaigns, prompts for practitioners to provide opportunistic reminders during consultations, practice strategies such as disease and vaccine registers to generate patient reminders (letters to patients and messages on repeat prescriptions advising influenza vaccination), more efficient vaccine supply and storage, better access through special clinics or home vaccination, together with benchmarking of practice performance and feedback to practices (Siriwardena, *et al.* 2003b; Siriwardena, *et al.* 2003a).

Effect of changes: outputs

We implemented these strategies in two studies. In a primary care trust study where we undertook an organisational intervention involving 32 of 39 practices, there were improvements in influenza vaccination rates in patients with heart disease (19%) and diabetes (17%) and those over 65 years of age (24%) (Siriwardena, *et al.* 2003b).

In a countywide study involving similar organisational interventions in 22 of

105 practices, there were significant improvements in vaccination rates in patients with heart disease (11%), diabetes (9%) and patients with a splenectomy (17%) (Siriwardena, *et al.* 2003a).

CONCLUSION

Quality improvement involves understanding and modifying processes of care to ensure that those processes that are critical to quality are delivered reliably, reducing unintended and unwanted variation. It is necessary to understand healthcare processes in order to improve them.

In this chapter, we have examined the use of the logic model to determine what information to collect from surveys, interviews, direct observations and other sources, and how to analyse this information using techniques such as process maps, critical-to-quality trees, driver diagrams and cause and effect diagrams, to design better and more reliable healthcare processes.

In the next chapter we will go on to look at the important issue of measurement and the use of statistical process control in determining to what extent, if any, improvement has occurred as a consequence of change in processes.

FURTHER READING

- Balestracci D (2006) Data 'sanity': statistics and reality. *Qual Prim Care.* **14**: 49–53.
- Balestracci D (2009) Quality in medical group practice – and for everyone: the importance of process. In: *Data sanity: a quantum leap to unprecedented results.* Medical Group Management Association: Englewood, NJ. pp. 1–12.

REFERENCES

Balestracci D (2009) *Data sanity: a quantum leap to unprecedented results.* Medical Group Management Association: Englewood, NJ.

Darzi of Denham AD (2008) *High quality care for all: NHS Next Stage Review final report.* CM 7432. The Stationery Office: London.

Deming WE (1982) *Out of the crisis.* Massachusetts Institute of Technology, Center for Advanced Engineering Study: Cambridge, MA.

Dexter LJ, Teare MD, Dexter M, *et al.* (2012) Strategies to increase influenza vaccination rates: outcomes of a nationwide cross-sectional survey of UK general practice. *BMJ Open.* **2**(3): e000851.

Dyas JV, Apekey TA, Tilling M, *et al.* (2010) Patients' and clinicians' experiences of consultations in primary care for sleep problems and insomnia: a focus group study. *Br J Gen Pract.* **60**(574): e180–200.

Iqbal M, Spaight PA, Siriwardena AN (2012) Patients' and emergency clinicians' perceptions of improving pre-hospital pain management: a qualitative study. *Emerg Med J.* Epub Apr 27.

Juran JM, Godfrey AB (1999) *Juran's quality handbook.* McGraw Hill: New York, NY.

Kyle SD, Morgan K, Spiegelhalder K, *et al.* (2011) No pain, no gain: an exploratory within-subjects mixed-methods evaluation of the patient experience of sleep restriction therapy (SRT) for insomnia. *Sleep Med.* **12**(8): 735–47.

Medeiros LC, Butkus SN, Chipman H, *et al.* (2005) A logic model framework for community nutrition education. *J Nutr Educ Behav.* **37**(4): 197–202.

Nolan T, Resar R, Haraden C, *et al.* (2013) *Improving the reliability of health care.* Institute for Healthcare Improvement: Cambridge, MA.

Siriwardena AN, Rashid A, Johnson M, *et al.* (2003a) Improving influenza and pneumococcal vaccination uptake in high-risk groups in Lincolnshire: a quality improvement report from a large rural county. *Qual Prim Care.* **11**: 19–28.

Siriwardena AN, Wilburn T, Hazelwood L (2003b) Increasing influenza and pneumococcal vaccination rates in high risk groups in one primary care trust. *Clin Gov.* **8**(3): 200–7.

Starfield B, Mangin D (2010) An international perspective on the basis for payment for performance. *Qual Prim Care.* **18**(6): 399–404.

CHAPTER 7

Measuring for improvement

SUMMARY

- Measurement is fundamental to knowing whether a change is an improvement and forms the 'study' aspect of the plan-do-study-act cycle.
- What we measure depends on what outcome we wish to achieve and therefore which parts of the process we should improve to do this.
- Measurement techniques such as run charts, control charts and funnel plots can help us to understand variation in healthcare processes, to assess whether processes are stable or improving and to determine how they can be improved further.
- Measurement itself is also a process that involves sources of possible variation.

INTRODUCTION

This chapter examines what to measure, how to measure it and techniques of measurement for improvement. As we learned in Chapter 6, everything we do can be seen as part of a process (Balestracci 2009). The structure (e.g. the equipment and materials used or the work environment), the processes of care (e.g. how people work and their work methods) and the outcomes of care are all important measures for evaluating quality (Donabedian 1966).

Measurement is itself a process that not only helps us to assess other processes but also can be used to drive improvement (Plsek 1999). The techniques for measurement that we discuss in this chapter will help us understand whether processes are stable, improving or deteriorating and the extent to which they can be improved further.

WHAT TO MEASURE

What we measure depends on what outcome we wish to achieve and therefore which parts of the process we should improve to do this. There are different types of measure. We can select particular criteria (also called audit or review criteria), standards and indicators (*see* also Chapter 5). The latter may include quality indicators, performance indicators or clinical performance indicators, depending on what is being measured and why.

A criterion (*see* also Chapter 5) is a measurable aspect of quality (structure, process or outcome) of care and has been defined as 'a systematically developed statement that can be used to assess the appropriateness of specific health-care decisions, services and outcomes' (Field and Lohr 1992). An example of a criterion is that every patient diagnosed with hypertension should have had his or her blood pressure recorded within the previous months. This is trans-lated into a measure: the proportion of patients with hypertension who have a blood pressure recorded within the previous 6 months (usually expressed as a percentage). If the criterion is based on research evidence that directly links it to improved outcomes, it is sometimes referred to as a 'review criterion'. For example, patients with hypertension should have a latest blood pressure read-ing (measured in the preceding 6 months) of 150/90 mmHg or less.

The level achieved for the criterion is compared with a standard – that is, what should be achieved. The standard is the threshold of expected compliance for the criterion. Standards are usually derived from consensus opinion (either local or from a wider group) or are based on a previous audit. Less commonly, a standard may be based on published evidence about levels of performance that lead to improved outcomes. An example here is the standard required to achieve herd immunity for measles, mumps and rubella vaccination of 95% of the population.

HOW TO MEASURE

Different types of improvement project use different types of measurement, but not all are equally useful or informative. Measurements are generally of three types: (1) before-and-after studies, (2) continuous assessments and (3) com-parative assessments.

Clinical audits characteristically employ before-and-after measurements where standards are compared before and after an intervention. The advantage of this approach is that it provides the analyst with a target to aim for and it is usually simple to analyse and present data. A disadvantage is that the stand-ard may be arbitrary. This may lead to gaming or unintended consequences. Furthermore, and most important, a change comparing a single measurement before and after an intervention may be an artefact of measurement rather than demonstrating a real improvement.

In contrast, quality improvement projects tend to use data that repeatedly measures processes over time. Data can be recorded as counts, rates or pro-portions (percentages). Rather than two measurements (i.e. before and after), multiple measurements are taken before, during and sometimes after the inter-vention has taken place. Relatively simple statistical methods are then used to analyse whether the process is showing a natural (or random) variation over time, and if so, can demonstrate the extent of this variation and whether real improvement (over and above natural variation) is occurring.

The advantage of this approach is that it helps us understand whether real improvement has taken place and it can demonstrate the extent of this improvement. It avoids interpreting natural variation as real change, and it ena-bles us to see the effects of multiple interventions over time. The disadvantage of this method is that measurements need to be taken repeatedly during the process of change and some basic analytical concepts and techniques need to be learned (*see* Table 7.1).

Measurement, whether using simple counts (e.g. numbers of referrals to hospital), rates (e.g. proportion of patients with a particular condition referred to hospital) or other more complex continuous variables, is also a process than can introduce variation. Data processes that include measurement, collection, analysis and interpretation – any or all of which may involve people, methods, machines, materials, 'measurements' (numbers) and environment as inputs – can also be a source of variation (Balestracci 2006). Therefore, it is important that data using samples or whole populations, ideally, for the purpose they were intended for are gathered, analysed and interpreted in a careful and consistent way.

Finally, we may wish to compare performance for different groups or organisations with the aim of comparing the best performers and the worst. The traditional method of doing this has been to represent performance of each organisation on a bar chart that ranks the highest with the lowest or vice versa. Unfortunately, this method can prevent a clear differentiation being made between the high-performing and low-performing organisations or groups. If they are aware of the method of presentation, it may lead them to aim for a middle rank in such a table, where they are less likely to be noticed. The pursuit of mediocrity can be prevented by using funnel plots to compare organisations. Funnel plots are a special type of control chart that compare different organisations rather than a single organisation over time.

TABLE 7.1 Measurement approaches in clinical audit and plan-do-study-act cycles

	Clinical audit	Plan-do-study-act
Criteria	Yes	Yes
Standards (target)	Yes	No
Type of measurement	Before-and-after	Continuous or repeated measurements over time (statistical process control)
Change implementation strategy	Change(s) are implemented after first audit (i.e. more rigid)	Multiple changes can be introduced in sequence or parallel (i.e. more flexible)
Cyclical	Yes	Yes
Ideal outcome	Meet or exceed standard	Improvement from baseline
Advantages	Simple to analyse	Analysis more complex
	Aims to achieve standard (target)	Aims to achieve improvement
Disadvantages	Does not account for natural (common cause) variation	Takes common cause variation into account
	Standard may be arbitrary	Improvement based on baseline performance rather than arbitrary standard

UNDERSTANDING VARIATION

Every measure of a process, a combination of processes or an outcome will show variation over time. Variation is therefore part of any process. It is inevitable, and ubiquitous, but it is amenable to measurement and control. If we want to demonstrate improvement, it is essential to select the key variables to measure quality in terms of outputs or outcomes that will signify improvement.

The natural variation of a stable process unaffected by the external factors affecting it or attempts to improve it is called 'common cause variation'. We see common cause variation in, for example, repeated measures of blood pressure. These may be due to changes in the physiological state of the individual, subtle differences in the technique of measurement or in the response to the measuring instrument.

For other measures, such as prescribing rates, these may vary over time due to differences in patient case mix between prescribers and in their prescribing behaviour. Similarly, referral rates, vaccination rates or, indeed, any other measure of health processes, organisations or systems will also vary over time because of variation in the process itself or in the process of measurement.

Variation that falls outside the 'common cause variation' is termed 'special cause variation'. As its name implies, 'special cause variation' is caused by an 'external' factor, whether this is planned or unplanned, intended or unintended. Analysing variation over time involves using statistical techniques, but the simplest way of analysing and representing such variation involves a technique called statistical process control, developed by Walter A Shewhart at Bell Telephone Laboratories in the 1920s (Mohammed, *et al.* 2001) and championed by W Edwards Deming (1982) and Joseph Juran (Juran, *et al.* 1974), Davis Balestracci (2009) and many others since. Table 7.2 summarises the differences between common and special cause variation.

TABLE 7.2 Differences between common and special cause variation

Common cause variation	Special cause variation
Is predictable	Unpredictable
Due to 'chance' causes	Due to 'assignable' causes
Many factors	Usually few factors
Often 'unknowable'	Can usually be identified
Is part of the process	Not part of the process
Affects process most of the time	Intermittently apparent

Any improvement in the healthcare process requires a change in a process to reduce the effect of 'common cause variation' and to trigger a 'special cause variation' that will represent a significant improvement. However, responding to common cause variation as though it is special cause variation has the opposite effect to that which is intended. It may actually increase the variation in the system. This is called 'tampering'. An example of tampering is when an organisation responds to a single reduction (or increase) in a measure *before* checking that the change is due to common cause variation.

Table 7.3 summarises how we should and should not respond to the different types of variation. A special cause strategy calls for investigation and explanation, which will sometimes lead to specific changes depending on the special cause identified. Common cause variation requires a different approach. A common cause strategy firstly requires us to explore the variation more closely using stratification to reveal any special causes. Next, one should seek to understand variation through the processes and systems that cause a problem. Finally, we should redesign processes to reduce inappropriate and unintended variation in an agreed measure in a way that is responsive to patients' needs (Siriwardena and Balestracci 2011).

TABLE 7.3 Responding to common and special cause variation

Common cause variation	Special cause variation
• Do not respond to individual results • Look at the average and the control limits • Understand reasons for common cause variation by looking at underlying processes and systems • Try to find special causes by stratification according to organisational unit • Improve the whole process if this is not acceptable or go for continuous quality improvement • Redesign processes to reduce inappropriate and unintended variation	• Respond appropriately to special cause variation • Investigate each point representing a special cause • Try to explain why the special cause has occurred and what factors led to it • Reinforce special causes leading to improvement while eliminating those leading to deterioration • Improve aspects of the process that have resulted in special cause variation • Redesign processes to reduce inappropriate and unintended variation

STATISTICAL PROCESS CONTROL
Run charts
Run charts are the simplest way of plotting data in chronological order. Data for a particular indicator are plotted as dots (data points) on a simple graph, with time plotted on the x-axis and the value of the indicator plotted on the y-axis. The time intervals should be ordered and sequential but not necessarily equal. They are often regularly spaced but need not be. At least 16 dots are usually required to see if a process is stable. The dots are connected by lines and a centre line, the median, is drawn. Figure 7.1 is a run chart showing hypnotic prescribing data for a single general practice.

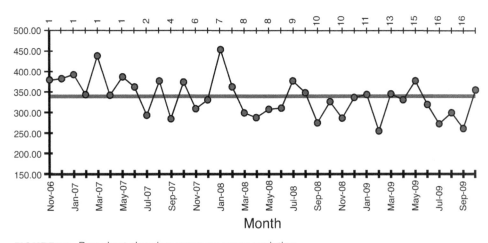

FIGURE 7.1 Run chart showing common cause variation

A 'run' is one or more data points above or below the median. Common cause variation is represented in a run chart as runs randomly distributed about the median. One way of conceptualising this is that in common cause variation the chance of a run being above or below the median is the same as the chance of throwing heads or tails with a coin. Three simple statistical rules have been developed to show whether there has been a significant change in a measure over time (i.e. a special cause variation).

These rules are helpful because they prevent individuals or groups just 'eyeballing' a chart of measurements over time and misinterpreting them. Following certain rules leads to consistent interpretation of what constitutes a significant change over time. This also prevents an inappropriate response to common cause variation as if it were a special cause.

The three rules that identify the most important types of special cause variation are shifts, trends and runs (shown in Box 7.1). A *shift* is a sequence or 'run' of seven dots above or below the median. An example of a shift is shown in Figure 7.2, which presents the rate of hypnotic drug prescribing in another general practice. The run chart shows a sequence of 25 dots. There are 11 dots below the median from January 2008, indicating a shift.

A *trend* is a sequence of seven dots all going upwards or downwards (dots on the same level are excluded from the count).

The final rule refers to *runs*, which give the 'run chart' its name. A 'run' is simply a sequence of dots above or below the median. Runs should be randomly distributed about the median when there is only common cause variation. Therefore, we can calculate if there are the right numbers of runs (between upper and lower limits) depending on how many dots there are in total in the chart, which gives a probability table for runs (*see* Table 7.4). In Figure 7.2 there are only four runs, when we would expect between 10 and 16 according to Table 7.4.

BOX 7.1 Basic rules for run charts

Run charts: a chronologically ordered sequence of data, with (usually at least 10) data points connected by lines and a centre (median) line. The following denote special causes.

- *Run:* a sequence of points either all above or all below the median
- *Shift:* seven or more successive data points above or below the median when there are up to 20 data points (eight or more with 20 or more data points)
- *Trend:* at seven (some experts accept six) or more data points going successively up or going down, including those on the median but not counting repeat values
- *Abnormal variability:* runs should be randomly distributed around the median, neither too few nor too many (*see* Table 7.2)
- *'Astronomical' data points:* there should not be any data points that are very obviously different from the rest of the data

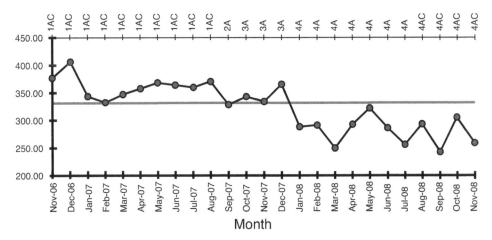

FIGURE 7.2 Run chart showing a 'shift'

TABLE 7.4 Probability table for runs

Number of observations (or dots)	Too few runs	Too many runs	Number of observations (or dots)	Too few runs	Too many runs
14	4	11			
15	4	12	28	10	19
16	5	12	29	10	20
17	5	13	30	11	21
18	6	13	31	11	21
19	6	14	32	11	22
20	6	15	33	11	22
21	7	15	34	12	23
22	7	16	35	13	23
23	8	16	36	13	24
24	8	17	37	13	25
25	9	17	38	14	25
26	9	18	39	14	26
27	9	19	40	15	26

Control charts

A control chart is a more sophisticated form of run chart. The relationship between a run chart and a control chart has been described as analogous to that between an X-ray and a magnetic resonance imaging scan (Carey 2003). The latter is more sensitive at detecting abnormalities but also more complex and requires greater resources. The principles of its construction and interpretation are very similar.

Figure 7.3 is a control chart showing hypnotic prescribing data for a single general practice and corresponding to the run chart in Figure 7.1. Again, data for a particular indicator are plotted as dots on a simple graph, with time plotted in chronological sequence on the x-axis and the value of the measurement or indicator of interest plotted on the y-axis. The time intervals should be sequential. They are often regularly spaced but need not be. The dots are connected by lines but this time the centre line is the mean line (*see* Figure 7.3).

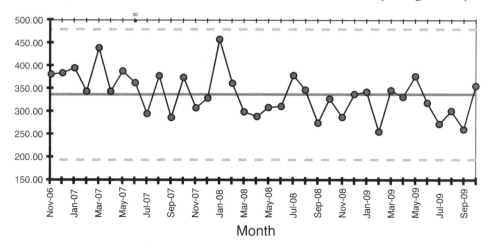

FIGURE 7.3 Control chart showing common cause variation

In addition, the control chart has two further lines: the upper and lower control (or sigma) limits, which define the variability in the data. They are different from confidence intervals or standard deviations and should not be confused with these. The control limits are lines also representing estimates of the dispersion or the boundaries in the data; standard deviations are used in specific charts of normally distributed physiological variables such as glucose or cholesterol. The mean and control limits should be calculated according to the population, sample size and type of data (i.e. the normal distribution for biological variables such as blood pressure, the Poisson distribution for count data, and the binomial distribution for yes/no or percentage performance data).

Confidence intervals are different from control limits. Confidence intervals are an estimate of the range of effect sizes around an odds ratio or risk ratio for a study. Confidence levels are usually set at 95%. Stated simply, this means that if a study were to be repeated 100 times, 95 times out of a 100 the effect size would fall between the 95% confidence intervals.

Common cause variation in a control chart is shown in Figure 7.3 (which shows the same data as the run chart in Figure 7.1). All the dots fall within the upper and lower control limits and are randomly distributed about the mean. Control charts are more sensitive at detecting significant change over time than run charts. There are more rules for determining significant changes over time in a control chart, but again four basic rules identify the most important types of special cause variation: a point outside the control limits, a shift, a trend and variability (*see* Box 7.2).

Figure 7.4 is a control chart showing hypnotic prescribing data for a single general practice corresponding to the run chart in Figure 7.2. In Figure 7.4

the second dot in the sequence falls above the upper control limit. A shift is a sequence of eight dots above or below the median (as shown in Figure 7.4). A trend is a sequence of six dots all going upwards or downwards (dots on the same level are again excluded from the count). A number of other rules can help to provide further signals that a significant change may have occurred. These are additional, more sensitive, rules but are also more likely to cause false positive signals and so they need to be interpreted with caution. This practice has significantly reduced its hypnotic drug prescribing since December 2007.

BOX 7.2 Basic rules for control charts

Control charts: a chronologically ordered sequence of at least 15–20 data points, with data points connected by lines, a centre (mean) line and upper and lower control limits. The following represent special causes.
- Single point outside the control limit
- *Shift:* eight or more data points above or below the mean
- *Trend:* at six or more data points going successively up or going down, including those on the mean but not counting repeat values
- *Abnormal variability:* two of three successive values more than two sigma limits from the mean

---

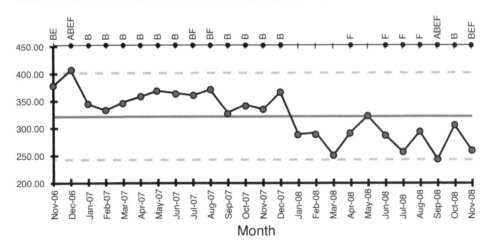

FIGURE 7.4 Control chart showing special causes

Funnel plots

As well as looking at an indicator across a period of time, control charts can also be used to compare organisational units at a single point or during a fixed period of time. In this type of control chart, organisational units are arranged on the x-axis with their performance as a count, rate or proportion (or percentage) on the y-axis. The mean is represented and control limits are calculated for each organisational unit based on all the data provided (*see* Figure 7.5).

In Figure 7.5 we represent data on the performance of ambulance stations as an organisational unit. In each case, a team of paramedics delivered care for patients with acute myocardial infarction (AMI) during a single month. Each dot represents an ambulance station. Performance is measured as the delivery of a process 'care bundle' for AMI. A care bundle is an all-or-none measure where every eligible patient with AMI should receive aspirin, glyceryl trinitrate, pain assessment and analgesia unless there is a valid exception. The delivery of the care bundle can vary from 0 to 1 (i.e. 0%–100%). The samples provided by each station were small, which led to wide control limits (0 and 1) for most stations. The mean performance was 44.4%, which meant that the care bundle was delivered to just over two out of every five patients.

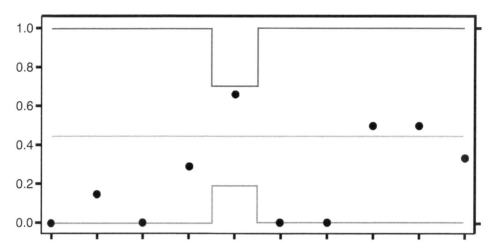

FIGURE 7.5 Control chart showing comparative (analysis of mean) performance for provision of care for acute myocardial infarction by ambulance station (P = mean probability = 0.44 [or 44%])

The control limits are denoted again by the outer lines which vary for each station. If data are arranged according to the size of the sample denominator provided by each organisational unit, this produces a funnel plot (*see* Figure 7.6).

In Figure 7.6 we see such a funnel plot showing AMI care bundle performance for 12 larger regional ambulance services in England. Each service is represented by a dot labelled between 1 and 12. The sample denominator is now greater but varies from a few cases (service 12) to over 200 cases (service 7) in the month that performance is measured. The mean performance across all the services is again around 45%.

The control limits that are now joined by a smooth line are wider for services with small samples of AMI and become narrower as the sample size increases. This produces the characteristic funnel shape of the control limits. Because this looks like the bell of a trombone, funnel plots are sometimes referred to as 'trombonograms'.

In the chart, one can immediately see that most trusts are contained within the control limits. The processes in these trusts deliver 'average' or common cause care defined by these control limits. Four trusts show performance either above or below the control limits. These trusts show significantly different performance, either higher or lower, than other trusts and this special cause requires

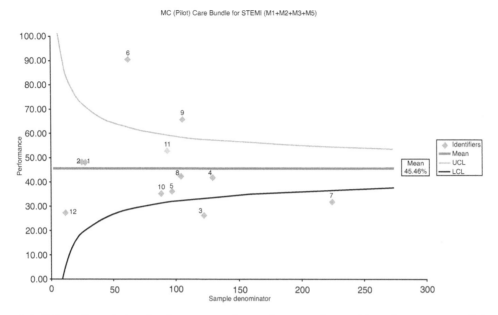

FIGURE 7.6 Funnel plot showing comparative performance for provision of acute myocardial care by ambulance services in England

further investigation to understand why this might be the case. The investigation may reveal a difference in the system of care providing this outcome.

CONCLUSION

This chapter has provided an introduction to measurement for improvement, a complex subject of growing importance. Repeated measurement over time is central to understanding variation in a process and how to improve quality. We have introduced readers to the principles of constructing and interpreting run and control charts and how to respond to common or special cause variation. Tomorrow's doctors and nurses will need to understand how the care they provide should be measured. This is a fast-changing field and more information on statistical process control is available from a number of excellent books, articles and online resources (*see* 'Further reading').

FURTHER READING

- Robert Lloyd (2014) *The science of improvement on a whiteboard!* Institute for Healthcare Improvement: Cambridge, MA. Available at: www.ihi.org/education/IHIOpenSchool/ resources/Pages/BobLloydWhiteboard.aspx#CC (accessed 26 April 2014).
- Balestracci D (2006) Statistics and reality: part 2. *Qual Prim Care.* **14**: 111–19.
- Mohammed MA (2004) Using statistical process control to improve the quality of health care. *Qual Saf Health Care.* **13**(4): 243–5.
- Mohammed MA, Worthington P, Woodall WH (2008) Plotting basic control charts: tutorial notes for healthcare practitioners. *Qual Saf Health Care.* **17**(2): 137–45.
- Stapenhurst T (2005) *Mastering statistical process control: a handbook for performance improvement using cases.* Butterworth-Heinemann: Oxford.

REFERENCES

Balestracci D (2006) Data 'sanity': statistics and reality. *Qual Prim Care.* **14**: 49–53.

Balestracci D (2009) *Data sanity: a quantum leap to unprecedented results.* Medical Group Management Association: Englewood, NJ.

Carey RG (2003) *Improving health care with control charts: basic and advanced SPC methods and case studies.* ASQ Quality Press: Milwaukee, WI.

Deming WE (1982) *Out of the crisis.* Massachusetts Institute of Technology, Center for Advanced Engineering Study: Cambridge, MA.

Donabedian A (1966) Evaluating the quality of medical care. *Milbank Mem Fund Q.* **44**(3 Suppl.): 166–206.

Field MJ, Lohr KN (1992) *Guidelines for clinical practice: from development to use.* The National Academies Press: Washington, DC.

Juran JM, Gryna FM, Bingham RS (1974) *Quality control handbook.* McGraw-Hill: New York, NY.

Mohammed MA, Cheng KK, Rouse A, *et al.* (2001) Bristol, Shipman, and clinical governance: Shewhart's forgotten lessons. *Lancet.* **357**(9254): 463–7.

Plsek PE (1999) Quality improvement methods in clinical medicine. *Pediatrics.* **103**(1 Suppl. E): 203–14.

Siriwardena AN, Balestracci D (2011) Using a common cause strategy for quality improvement: improving hypnotic prescribing in general practice within a quality improvement collaborative. *Qual Prim Care.* **19**(5): 283–7.

CHAPTER 8

Systems, safety and spread

SUMMARY

- The healthcare system describes a complex interacting network of healthcare staff, organisations and technologies.
- Positive change in health systems depends on these interactions.
- A focus on systems can help to design strategies for better and safer healthcare that are less reliant on individual actions and effort.
- Successful improvement and its spread requires an understanding of the system, including the context for improvement, the networks and interactions involved and an understanding of how to deal with complexity.

INTRODUCTION

In your working lifetime, how much more complex has the practice of primary care become? The shift of most diabetes care into the community provides a conspicuous example. How many different players and processes now contribute to the comprehensive care of chronic diseases? We accept as axiomatic the need to 'integrate' different elements of healthcare to form a coherent whole. In this chapter we describe health systems, how they work, why they respond to change in unexpected ways and how this knowledge can be used to bring about safer care and spread improvement.

HEALTHCARE SYSTEMS

A system is a set of interdependent and interacting elements or actors, together with the context in which they operate, that seeks to achieve a common aim. In broad terms, healthcare systems may be considered in terms of size and complexity as macro-level (healthcare organisations interacting at a geographical, regional or national level), meso-level (healthcare organisations themselves) or micro-level (groups of clinical and/or non-clinical staff working together within an organisation or a healthcare setting) – so-called clinical microsystems.

Clinical microsystems comprise groups of clinicians interacting to provide specific types of care for patients. The clinical microsystem is made up of the actors in the system, how they relate to their patients and one another, and the context in which they do this. Contextual factors include regulation, payments and resources, leadership, culture, training, capability and aims or targets (Kaplan, *et al.* 2012). The design of the healthcare *system* can profoundly affect quality of care, more so than the individuals or elements of care from which the system is formed.

This leads to the oft-repeated adage of health systems experts, that 'every system is perfectly designed to get the results it achieves' (Nolan 1998). Much more than individual workers in the system, it is the design of the health system that is critical to its success or failure – and for improvement to occur attention needs to be paid to the system and its (re)design.

Interactions within these complex socio-technical (human-behavioural-health technology) systems (Braithwaite, *et al.* 2009) are an important feature and are governed by mathematical laws: the laws of natural networks (Barabási and Albert 1999).

Point to ponder
- How would you describe the healthcare system you work in, what are the key components and where are the critical interactions?

NETWORKS AND COMPLEXITY

Natural networks can be conceptualised as a web, with individuals or organisations as vertices (the points where lines intersect) and social interactions as edges (of these lines). The model states that networks expand continuously by adding new vertices, and these new vertices attach preferentially to others that are already well connected, so-called nodes; with very large numbers of connections these nodes are termed hubs. Healthcare and other groups of interacting actors are predicted to develop as a characteristic of these principles (Ravasz and Barabási 2003).

Natural networks often behave in unpredictable ways: the boundaries of these networks are vague or fuzzy because members of a network often interact or are associated with other groups or organisations; the individuals and groups adapt and co-evolve with others in response to a variety of stimuli; their actions are often based on tacit internalised rules as well as explicit ones.

The complex interactions within and between natural networks can also lead to novel behaviours in response to external forces. This is because responses to various stimuli are often non-linear and unpredictable rather than a simple linear cause and effect reactions (Plsek and Greenhalgh 2001). Different types of intervention (tools, communication, behaviours, and so forth) rather than simple levers need to be employed to influence networks: these are sometimes called 'attractor patterns' because they involve more subtle efforts at attracting rather than directing behaviour change (Plsek and Wilson 2001; Thaler and Sunstein 2008).

The characteristics of networks within complex systems, which include aspects such as self-organisation, weak interactions and informal communications, are beginning to be understood (Cunningham, *et al.* 2011). The central nodes or hubs in natural networks are opinion leaders; these key individuals are often but not always in leadership positions, but they are always better connected, have greater influence on others and are therefore important as change agents. Communication in natural networks is predominantly informal rather than formal; messages that are heard and conveyed by recipients are those that have natural appeal and are termed 'sticky'.

For more complex information to be accessible and sticky, it needs to be organised and simplified into natural categories or maps. Such information eventually becomes part of the collective knowledge reaching a natural 'tipping point', where it is so well diffused that it becomes sufficient to be acted on (Braithwaite, *et al.* 2009).

There are various barriers and facilitators to communication between networks and their members, such as professional identity, organisational culture, homophily (attraction to those who are similar to us in various attributes) and communication style (Braithwaite 2010).

An example of a healthcare network is a clinical community focused on quality improvement, such as the quality improvement collaborative. The ideas of complex systems and natural networks help to explain why some collaboratives work better than others in bringing about improvement and innovation (Siriwardena 2012).

Point to ponder

● Think about an innovation you would like to implement. What are the barriers and facilitators relating to the innovation, the professionals involved and the organisational culture in which it is to be implemented?

IMPROVING SAFETY

Systems thinking has revolutionised the way we think about improving safety in healthcare. Rather than considering errors as being due to individual mistakes, lessons from the aviation and other industries show that errors are often built into the design of healthcare systems and processes. Reason's well-known 'Swiss cheese model' shows how major errors can arise from multiple small defects (the 'holes' in the cheese) in the existing system of care (Reason 2000). These errors might be averted by understanding where these small defects might occur and by putting in further safeguards to prevent them.

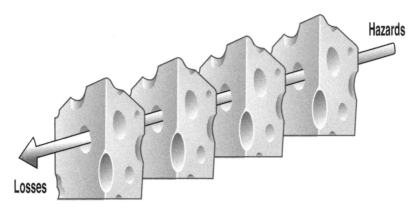

FIGURE 8.1 The Swiss cheese model of error (Reason 2000)

One way of systematically detecting, quantifying and classifying errors is through the use of 'trigger tools'; these are instruments developed to measure the rate of harm or changes in harm using a structured record review in a variety of healthcare settings (Resar, *et al.* 2003). Another method is reviewing malpractice claims. In primary care, claims are most commonly due to delayed or missed diagnoses and prescribing errors (Wallace, *et al.* 2013).

A better understanding of when and where diagnostic errors might occur and why these might lead to delays in treatment can help to reduce these failures. For example, greater knowledge of common prescribing errors (Thomas, *et al.* 2013; Avery, *et al.* 2011) can allow prompts and reminders linked to prescribing safety indicators to be integrated into computer systems (Kuperman, *et al.* 2007).

Serious errors, whether these might occur in a community or acute setting, are designated as 'never events', defined as 'serious, largely preventable patient safety incidents that should not occur if the available preventative measures have been implemented by health care provider' (NHS Commissioning Board 2013). Examples of 'never events' include wrong-site surgery; serious medication errors, such as daily rather than weekly administration of methotrexate (NHS England 2014); or failure to refer a patient suspected of having cancer (de Wet, *et al.* 2014). Systematic measures to prevent 'never events' can help to provide healthcare more safely.

> **Point to ponder**
> ● Think about a recent error in your practice. What systematic measures could be put in place to prevent this occurring?

SPREADING INNOVATION AND IMPROVEMENT

Greenhalgh, *et al.* (2004) have defined innovation in service delivery and organisation as:

> a novel set of behaviours, routines, and ways of working that are directed at improving health outcomes, administrative efficiency, cost effectiveness, or users' experience and that are implemented by planned and coordinated actions.

Fundamental to change is the management of people and an understanding of how they will react is invaluable.

We can spread innovation using passive approaches (diffusion), active efforts directed at a target group (dissemination), wider efforts covering entire organisations (implementation) and finally achieving normalisation where an innovation is so embedded that it is no longer an innovation but routinised into practice (Greenhalgh, *et al.* 2004).

The model of spread developed by Greenhalgh and based on Rogers's seminal work on diffusion of innovations (Rogers 2003; *see also* Chapter 2 Figure 2.1) provides a comprehensive model of how spread can occur. It shows how innovations can spread depending on the innovation itself, the organisational system(s), the external context, individual actors, the interactions between these (communication, influence and linkages) and the consequences of adoption or assimilation (Greenhalgh, *et al.* 2004).

Depending on their structural characteristics, the networks that support spread are motivated by two contrasting and sometimes competing functions: first, in structurally dense networks, characterised by high degrees of interconnectedness, they provide safety and affiliation through a web of close trusting relationships; second, networks – particularly those with segments having less-dense connections and more structural holes – enable nodes (agents) that span these segments to facilitate the flow of information. The ability to link segments through conveying knowledge or providing a communication channel also increases the effectiveness and enhances the status of these agents. Agents that can perform this function are sometimes called 'boundary spanners', 'mavens', 'salesmen', 'connectors' or 'brokers': they are the change agents that enable diffusion and spread of ideas (Siriwardena and Gillam 2014).

Traditionally, networks in healthcare are based on professional groups or organisations. This reflects how health professionals are trained and how they are employed. Professional and organisational boundaries often constitute structural holes, where gaps in care are evident at the interfaces between groups and organisations (Braithwaite 2010). Improvement initiatives – for example, quality improvement collaboratives (Siriwardena, *et al.* 2014) – provide a real opportunity for healthcare staff in a variety of professional groups and across organisational boundaries to learn about quality improvement methods and to apply these to gaps in the care they provide (Cunningham, *et al.* 2011).

Change agents affect the early stages of diffusion through three modes of influence: (1) they can be a direct source of advice, (2) they can seek to actively persuade or (3) they can provide a model to be followed. This latter is often termed 'opinion leadership'. Opinion leaders within organisations characteristically have slightly higher status, have greater degrees of connectedness and have more personal influence than their followers or others in their network. Rather than being innovators or early adopters, they are usually found in the early majority on the adoption curve.

Adoption is the result of a number of factors including the appeal or 'stickiness' of the idea itself; the effect of advice, persuasion or modelling by change agents; and the effect of external influences to overcome resistance to change. The early, slower phase of adoption is usually the result of persuasion and external influence. The more rapid, mid-phase of adoption occurs when adoption accelerates through modelling or imitation without persuasion or external influence, and this is sometimes termed the 'tipping point', at which innovations become adopted very widely (Gladwell 2002).

These ideas and principles can be used to further spread innovations including quality improvement initiatives. Spreading improvement from a successful local initiative to wider implementation involves careful preparation, agreeing aims, developing a spread plan and implementing the plan (Massoud, *et al.* 2006).

Preparation involves understanding the system, its context, and in particular the organisational leadership and its readiness for change. The aim for spread should include the organisations and people, the improvement goals and measures, and the time period for implementation.

Implementation of spread needs consideration of the steps by which this will occur and what the facilitators and barriers may be, including existing organisational support, structures and culture for change, what changes need to be made to these to effect spread and how changes can be normalised into practice (Massoud, *et al.* 2006).

BOX 8.1 Case study – spreading improvement in influenza and pneumococcal vaccination uptake

This study began with work in a single general practice looking at facilitators and barriers of vaccination uptake (Siriwardena 1999). The knowledge of these enablers and blockers together with evidence on what factors were most likely to lead to change (e.g. protocols, reminders to patient and staff, registers) were gathered from patients and staff, and this was shared and applied in a large primary care organisation to an organisational collaborative involving 32 (of 39) practices. General practices were attracted to participate because there were national guidelines supported by good evidence for influenza vaccination, they were already undertaking a vaccination programme, there was remuneration for vaccination, which compensated for the additional costs of improving the vaccination programme, and there was support provided through a primary care organisation (the Clinical Audit Advisory Group).

This led to improvements in vaccine rates in patients with heart disease (19% increase in influenza vaccination; 15% increase in pneumococcal vaccination), patients with diabetes (17% increase in influenza vaccination; 13% increase in pneumococcal vaccination) and patients over 65 years of age (24% increase in influenza vaccination) (Siriwardena, *et al.* 2003b). We can calculate the likely benefits of this intervention. Assuming 1000 patients were eligible for vaccination in each practice, with an average of three general practitioners (GPs) per practice, and a change of 20% in vaccination rate in 39 practices, this equates to an additional 6400 patients vaccinated, and over 60 GPs and their staff involved during the course of this study. The number needed to treat to prevent one death is 120, which meant that around 50 deaths would have been prevented through this intervention.

A further collaborative involving a similar organisational intervention in 22 of 105 practices in one county led to significant improvements in vaccine rates in patients with heart disease (11% increase in influenza vaccination; 28% increase in pneumococcal vaccination), patients with diabetes (9% increase in influenza vaccination; 29% increase in pneumococcal vaccination) and patients with a splenectomy (17% increase in influenza vaccination; 16% increase in pneumococcal vaccination). There were again over 60 GPs involved, with approximately 4400 additional patients receiving influenza and pneumococcal vaccination, and prevention of around 37 deaths as well as hospitalisations (Siriwardena, *et al.* 2003a).

The ideas were formally tested in a randomised controlled trial of a complex intervention to improve influenza and pneumococcal vaccination rates in 30 practices and this also showed positive effects for pneumococcal vaccination (Siriwardena, *et al.* 2002). A subsequent cross-sectional study, investigating factors associated with success of practice seasonal influenza vaccination campaigns, showed strategies that if widely implemented by general practices would improve average influenza vaccination rates by 7%–8% (Dexter, *et al.* 2012).

These strategies have been spread more widely by being introduced into the national UK influenza vaccination campaigns of 2012/13 and 2013/14 (Department of Health 2013; Department of Health 2012).

The mechanisms of spread have included small-scale testing, leading to large-scale collaborative interventions supported by education, audit and feedback and national guidance.

(Siriwardena 2003)

CONCLUSION

Healthcare systems that include people, organisations and health technologies are perfectly designed to get the results they achieve. Improvements in processes, outcomes and safety depend on the complex interactions between people and health technologies, and a better understanding of these can help design better healthcare systems and successfully spread improvement.

FURTHER READING

- Darzi of Denham AD (2008) *High quality care for all: NHS Next Stage Review final report.* CM 7432. The Stationery Office: London.
- Donaldson L (2000) *An organisation with a memory: report of an expert group on learning from adverse events in the NHS chaired by the Chief Medical Officer.* The Stationery Office: London.

REFERENCES

Avery AJ, Dex GM, Mulvaney C, *et al.* (2011) Development of prescribing-safety indicators for GPs using the RAND Appropriateness Method. *Br J Gen Pract.* 61(589): e526–36.

Barabási AL, Albert R (1999) Emergence of scaling in random networks. *Science.* 286(5439): 509–12.

Braithwaite J (2010) Between-group behaviour in health care: gaps, edges, boundaries, disconnections, weak ties, spaces and holes. A systematic review. *BMC Health Serv Res.* 10: 330.

Braithwaite J, Runciman WB, Merry AF (2009) Towards safer, better healthcare: harnessing the natural properties of complex sociotechnical systems. *Qual Saf Health Care.* 18(1): 37–41.

Cunningham FC, Ranmuthugala G, Plumb J, *et al.* (2011) Health professional networks as a vector for improving healthcare quality and safety: a systematic review. *BMJ Qual Saf.* Epub Nov 30.

Department of Health (2013) *The flu immunisation programme 2013/14.* Department of Health: London.

Department of Health (2012) *Seasonal flu plan: winter 2012/13.* HMSO: London.

De Wet C, O'Donnell C, Bowie P (2014) Developing a preliminary 'never event' list for general practice using consensus-building methods. *Br J Gen Pract.* 64(620): e159–67.

Dexter LJ, Teare MD, Dexter M, *et al.* (2012) Strategies to increase influenza vaccination rates: outcomes of a nationwide cross-sectional survey of UK general practice. *BMJ Open.* 2(3): e000851.

Gladwell M (2002) *The tipping point: how little things can make a big difference.* Back Bay Books: Boston, MA.

Greenhalgh T, Robert G, Macfarlane F, *et al.* (2004) Diffusion of innovations in service organizations: systematic review and recommendations. *Milbank Q.* 82(4): 581–629.

Kaplan HC, Provost LP, Froehle CM, *et al.* (2012) The Model for Understanding Success in Quality (MUSIQ): building a theory of context in healthcare quality improvement. *BMJ Qual Saf.* 21(1): 13–20.

Kuperman GJ, Bobb A, Payne TH, *et al.* (2007) Medication-related clinical decision support in computerized provider order entry systems: a review. *J Am Med Inform Assoc.* 14(1): 29–40.

Massoud MR, Nielsen GA, Nolan K, *et al.* (2006) *A framework for spread: from local improvements to system-wide change.* Institute for Healthcare Improvement: Cambridge, MA.

NHS Commissioning Board (2013) *Serious Incident Framework March 2013: an update to the 2010 National Framework for Reporting and Learning from Serious Incidents Requiring Investigation.* Department of Health: London.

NHS England (2014) *The never events list 2013/14 update.* Department of Health: London.

Nolan TW (1998) Understanding medical systems. *Ann Intern Med.* **128**(4): 293–8.

Plsek PE, Greenhalgh T (2001) Complexity science: the challenge of complexity in health care. *BMJ.* **323**(7313): 625–8.

Plsek PE, Wilson T (2001) Complexity, leadership, and management in healthcare organisations. *BMJ.* **323**(7315): 746–9.

Ravasz E, Barabási AL (2003) Hierarchical organization in complex networks. *Phys Rev E Stat Nonlin Soft Matter Phys.* **67**(2 Pt. 2): 026112.

Reason J (2000) Human error: models and management. *BMJ.* **320**(7237): 768–70.

Resar RK, Rozich JD, Classen D (2003) Methodology and rationale for the measurement of harm with trigger tools. *Qual Saf Health Care.* **12**(Suppl. 2): ii39–45.

Rogers EM (2003) *Diffusion of innovations.* 5th ed. Free Press: New York, NY.

Siriwardena AN (2012) Why quality improvement initiatives succeed or fail: the MUSIQ of quality improvement. *Qual Prim Care.* **20**(1): 1–3.

Siriwardena AN (2003) *The impact of educational interventions on influenza and pneumococcal vaccination rates in primary care.* De Montfort University: Leicester.

Siriwardena AN (1999) Targeting pneumococcal vaccination to high-risk groups: a feasibility study in one general practice. *Postgrad Med J.* **75**(882): 208–12.

Siriwardena AN, Gillam S (2014) Systems and spread. *Qual Prim Care.* **22**(1): 7–10.

Siriwardena AN, Rashid A, Johnson M, *et al.* (2003a) Improving influenza and pneumococcal vaccination uptake in high-risk groups in Lincolnshire: a quality improvement report from a large rural county. *Qual Prim Care.* **11**: 19–28.

Siriwardena AN, Rashid A, Johnson MR, *et al.* (2002) Cluster randomised controlled trial of an educational outreach visit to improve influenza and pneumococcal immunisation rates in primary care. *Br J Gen Pract.* **52**(482): 735–40.

Siriwardena AN, Shaw D, Essam N, *et al.* (2014) The effect of a national quality improvement collaborative on prehospital care for acute myocardial infarction and stroke in England. *Implement Sci.* **9**: 17.

Siriwardena AN, Wilburn T, Hazelwood L (2003b) Increasing influenza and pneumococcal vaccination rates in high risk groups in one primary care trust. *Clin Gov.* **8**: 200–7.

Thaler RH, Sunstein CR (2008) *Nudge: improving decisions about health, wealth, and happiness.* Yale University Press: New Haven, CT.

Thomas SK, McDowell SE, Hodson J, *et al.* (2013) Developing consensus on hospital prescribing indicators of potential harms amenable to decision support. *Br J Clin Pharmacol.* **76**(5): 797–809.

Wallace E, Lowry J, Smith SM, *et al.* (2013) The epidemiology of malpractice claims in primary care: a systematic review. *BMJ Open.* **3**(7): e002929.

CHAPTER 9

Financial incentives

SUMMARY

- Pay for performance can make an important contribution to improving quality of care but needs to be considered in the context of other motivating factors.
- UK general practices receive substantial financial rewards for achieving standards set out in the Quality and Outcomes Framework (QOF).
- Observed improvements in quality of care for chronic diseases in the framework have been modest, and the impact on costs, professional behaviour and patient experience remains uncertain.
- However, differences in performance between deprived and non-deprived areas have lessened.
- Understanding of the QOF, forward planning and good organisation are essential to achieve a practice's maximum QOF potential.

INTRODUCTION

Introduced in 2004, the UK Quality and Outcomes Framework (QOF) is the most comprehensive national primary care pay-for-performance (P4P) scheme in the world (Roland 2004). The QOF is more than a payment scheme: it is a complex intervention comprising a number of elements including financial incentives and information technology (computerised prompts and decision support) that is designed to promote structured and team-based care with the aim of achieving evidence-based quality targets.

It was one component in the reorganisation of primary care resulting from a new General Medical Services contract for general practitioners (GPs), which led to a practice-based, rather than practitioner-based, contract, and investment to reward quality of care through both fixed and performance-related funding streams. The financial incentives are substantial, with a maximum of 1000 points available to practices, and an average payment per practice in 2013–14 of £133.76 for each point achieved.

Over half of these points are allocated to clinical indicators, which currently cover 20 chronic conditions. In 2012–13, practices in England achieved an average of 960.8 points (or 96.1%). However, for 2014–15, the QOF is being scaled back by over one-third, to a total of 559 points (Health and Social Care Information Centre 2013).

A recent Cochrane Review found that, while P4P schemes improved patients' well-being, the effects of financial incentive schemes on the quality of primary healthcare were 'modest and variable' (Scott, *et al.* 2011). The huge variation in P4P schemes in different countries has made it difficult for reviewers to draw generalisable conclusions, whereas the uniform design of the QOF lends itself to close scrutiny. The research evidence about the QOF has thus grown rapidly.

As the QOF payment forms a significant proportion of practice income, it is important for practices to achieve maximum points as efficiently as possible. This involves detailed knowledge of the QOF process, up-to-date awareness of QOF targets and the changes that are made to these year on year, forward planning, and clear mechanisms within the practice to achieve these targets.

We undertook the first systematic review examining the impact of the QOF on the quality of UK primary medical care (Gillam, *et al.* 2012). This chapter looks at what we have learned about the use of financial incentives and how to manage them effectively at practice level.

HOW HAS THE QUALITY AND OUTCOMES FRAMEWORK IMPROVED QUALITY OF CARE?

The implementation of the QOF has helped consolidate evidence-based practice. It has been associated with an increased rate of improvement of quality of care over the first year of implementation, returning to pre-intervention rates of improvement in subsequent years. There have been modest reductions in mortality and hospital admissions in some areas (Shohet, *et al.* 2007), and where it has been assessed, these modest improvements appear cost-effective (Walker, *et al.* 2010). The QOF has led to narrowing of differences in performance between deprived and non-deprived areas (Doran, *et al.* 2008a). It has strengthened team-working.

The knock-on effect of the QOF in unincentivised areas has been disappointing (Doran, *et al.* 2011). Prescription rates for antidepressants, statins and other drugs have risen but this is not clearly attributable to the QOF. The costs of administering the scheme are substantial (£1 billion per year), and some staff are concerned that primary care has become more biomedical in focus and less patient centred.

The QOF has strengthened team-working and promoted a diversity of new roles especially for nurses (McGregor, *et al.* 2008). Indeed, the QOF may have diminished the workload of GPs, enabling them to concentrate on more complex care, and led to teams in which work and knowledge is more evenly distributed among its members.

The QOF has been described as 'scientific bureaucratic medicine' where indicators and guidelines are perceived as threatening professionalism in various ways (Checkland and Harrison 2010). For better or worse, the QOF can be seen to have reduced clinical autonomy and to have provided performance data that can be used to compare providers nationally.

Remarkably little is known of what patients make of these changes, although anecdotal reports point to unintended consequences detracting from patient-centred care (Wilkie 2010). The fear expressed by some that adherence to single disease-based guidelines might override respect for patient autonomy, lead clinicians to ignore co-morbidities, promote a mechanistic approach to chronic disease management, or reduce clinical practice to a series of dichotomised decisions at the expense of personal aspects of care is not borne out by the research to date.

Several factors impair the QOF's impact at population level. Setting targets below 100% and the process of 'exception reporting' reduces the public health effectiveness of population targets by shifting the focus of the practice away from harder-to-reach patients. More fundamentally, payment for adhering to guidelines cannot be assumed to improve health status, regardless of whether it improves performance. This is because improved processes (e.g. treating hypertension) may not always translate to improved outcomes (e.g. stroke prevention), because of other powerful confounding influences on outcomes such as differential access to care, non-modifiable risk factors (genetics, familial) or patterns of co-morbidity. Process measures are often preferred for incentive schemes, as they are under the control of the health system and can be more efficient (Mant and Hicks 1995). The QOF's evidence base will only ever be partial, because its indicators by their very nature will focus on measuring the measurable.

DEVELOPING P4P IN THE UNITED KINGDOM

The limited evidence for the scheme's cost-effectiveness is a central critique for the QOF's detractors. If £1 billion a year of additional funding to general practice has yielded only modest improvements in measured quality of care, might greater benefits have been achieved if this investment had funded an alternative approach to quality improvement? The opportunity costs of the QOF are to a great extent unknowable but the imperfect evidence available suggests that the same benefits could be maintained at reduced cost, particularly if systems are designed to involve clinicians and align with their values (Marshall and Harrison 2005).

Although some have argued for discarding the QOF, it seems wiser to concentrate on addressing weaknesses rather than throwing away the gains. There is no reason why both technical aspects of quality and personal care cannot improve together (Gillam and Siriwardena 2010). The involvement of the National Institute for Health and Care Excellence has greatly strengthened the QOF's scientific underpinnings. There will always be a fine judgement about timing, level of evidence required and whether to accept a consensus rather than an evidence-based indicator. The evidence base for existing indicators needs to be under constant review. Some indicators for which performance has reached a ceiling may need to be retired, although performance may not be maintained (Reeves, *et al.* 2010).

Gaming is known to occur in many systems that are driven by pay for performance. However, there has been little evidence of gaming in the QOF despite, or perhaps because of, a rigorous system of checks at various levels. On the contrary, practices are exceeding the upper payment thresholds and levels of exception reporting continue to fall year on year (Doran, *et al.* 2008b). Nevertheless, vigilant monitoring systems are needed. The balance of fixed versus performance-related funding should be reviewed. There is merit in linking the size of financial rewards to the public health impact of attaining individual indicators (Fleetcroft, *et al.* 2010).

Future developments need their own evidence base and there is a clear need for more experimental research. Does the size of incentive payments affect achievement? How can the patient experience be assessed better, and more directly linked to the payment of financial incentives? Do incentives lead to a trade-off between technical and patient-centred dimensions of quality, or can they produce improvements across different dimensions of quality? What effect do incentives have on harder-to-measure outcomes such as the interpersonal aspects of care, and care for underserved populations? What is the optimum time for a quality indicator to be included in a payment scheme before being reviewed or replaced by a different incentive?

In recognition of some of its limitations, the QOF is being scaled down in the coming year.

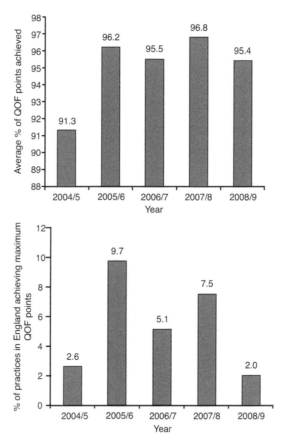

FIGURE 9.1 Quality and Outcomes Framework achievement for English practices, 2004–09 (*data source:* NHS Information Centre for Health and Social Care)

TRANSFORMING PRACTICE

The QOF has changed staffing structures and working practices. The bulk of the clinical points within the QOF are available for chronic disease management, and most of the work to achieve these points is performed by practice nurses, using disease registers and call–recall systems. They work with protocols and disease-specific chronic disease management templates, in practice-based chronic disease management clinics.

Although potentially efficient, there are problems associated with this model of care. Especially in larger practices where a single nurse often specialises in a single disease area, practices nurses and GPs can become deskilled. For example, patients with several chronic medical problems can be invited to three or four separate clinics if the nurses running these clinics are not skilled to perform all the disease checks required in a single appointment.

The QOF has also increased the number of administrative staff within most practices. Even quite small practices may employ someone simply to ensure the smooth running of QOF. Finally, of course, QOF has dramatically increased practice workload.

OPTIMISING QUALITY AND OUTCOMES FRAMEWORK ATTAINMENTS

Box 9.1 summarises ways that practices can increase their QOF points (Simon and Morton 2010).

BOX 9.1 Top 10 tips for obtaining Quality and Outcomes Framework points

1   Know the rules
2   Plan your strategy at the start of the year
3   Work at your QOF targets all year
4   Involve the whole team
5   Use your practice computer system effectively
6   Actively target specific patient groups
7   Maximise points for patients on multiple disease registers
8   Scrutinise exception reporting
9   Think laterally
10   Link QOF to other practice activities

Know the rules
The QOF is under continual review and updates are introduced at intervals. It is important to know what is required for each standard. Invest in training where necessary.

Plan your strategy at the start of the year
Planning is essential to maximise QOF income. It is too late to do much about unmet targets if failure to achieve the required standards is flagged too late in the year. Prior to the start of the financial year, meet to look at changes to the QOF from the previous year, such as new standards required. Target the processes and QOF domains identified for improvement and assign responsibility for each QOF area to a member of the clinical team.

Work at your QOF targets all year
Ensure regular internal interim QOF reviews. If the practice is falling behind on one standard then have a drive to increase achievement levels.

Involve the whole team

The income generated by the QOF affects the whole practice. All staff, including receptionists and administration staff, should take responsibility for achieving the maximum QOF points available (*see* Box 9.2). Consider staff training sessions, reviewing job descriptions and changing induction procedures to ensure staff understand why maximising QOF achievement is important and what their roles are. Consider performance-related pay or bonuses for key staff such as the practice manager for delivering improved QOF achievement.

BOX 9.2 Case study – involving the team

The Copse Surgery noticed as the year end approaches that the percentage of patients aged over 15 years whose notes record 'never smoked' or smoking status in the past 27 months was only 76%. Dr Green was dispatched to deal with the problem.

He asked the computer manager to add a prompt to flash up on screen whenever any patient's notes without a smoking status record, or with a record added more than a year previously of the patient being a smoker or ex-smoker, were accessed. He asked all of those in direct patient contact (doctors, nurses and reception staff) to ask patients their smoking status if they spotted the prompt box and put a large notice up in each consulting room to remind clinical staff. He also asked the repeat prescribing clerk to attach a letter to repeat prescriptions, asking patients without a recent smoking status or 'never smoked' record to let the practice know whether and how much they smoke.

Two weeks later he reviewed the situation. Although the percentage had gone up to 79% there was still some way to go to reach the 90% target. Checking a random sample of patients without a recent record, he noted that most were not regular attenders at the surgery. It was therefore difficult to target them via direct encounters. He proposed two evening telephone sessions when receptionists were paid to come in to ring all those on the list of patients with no recent record of smoking status. The proposal was approved. After 4 frantic hours of telephoning, the percentage was up to 90.8%.

Afterwards there was a meeting to discuss what went wrong. Several factors emerged. Many of the patients recorded as ex-smokers on the computer had only tried one or two cigarettes ever. It was agreed that these patients should be recoded as non-smokers and then, once over the age of 25, will not need to be asked their smoking status every 27 months. Everyone also agreed that next year's smoking data should be collected throughout the year, especially for new registrations and when infrequent attenders come to the surgery.

Use your practice computer effectively

All licensed GP software includes mechanisms to record QOF data. It is important to ensure that the correct Read codes are entered to enable the computer to extract all relevant information. Every system does this slightly differently, so it is important to ensure that everyone entering data is aware of the terms and templates they should be using on your system.

Actively target specific patient groups

Targeting specific patient groups is integral to the achievement of maximum QOF points. Make sure that your chronic disease registers are accurate. Wrongly diagnosed and thus untreated patients will count against your percentage achievement. It is also important to ensure that regular reviews take place and that all data required are recorded at each review, using templates and reminders to ensure that nothing is missed. If disease prevalence is lower than average, the practice will lose points value through prevalence adjustments, so it is important to ensure that patients with chronic diseases are included on disease registers. If prevalence is still low, target high-risk groups to ensure that patients with these chronic diseases are not being missed.

Maximise points for patients on multiple disease registers

Many patients have multiple chronic diseases. For example, it is not uncommon for a single individual to be obese, a smoker, have coronary heart disease, chronic obstructive pulmonary disease, chronic kidney disease, diabetes mellitus and a history of stroke. It is important to make sure that reviews for these multiple-category patients take place, as missing reviews can affect multiple targets. There are many common elements in the reviews required for several of the domains, so combining routine reviews for all the conditions affecting that patient is both a cost- and time-effective way of maximising QOF points.

Scrutinise exception reporting

The QOF includes the concept of 'exception reporting'. This was introduced so that practices were not penalised where, for example, patients do not attend for review, or where a medication cannot be prescribed because of a contraindication or side effect.

The overall exception rate for England, across all indicator groups, is just over 5%. Look at your practice exception rate compared with national and local figures. If you are excepting too many patients, check that you can justify your exceptions (*see* Box 9.3).

BOX 9.3 Case study – exception reporting

Jane, the nurse running the cardiovascular clinic in the Beech Practice, had a big push to review patients with heart failure. She was disappointed when told that she had fallen just short of the maximum points target for the percentage on an angiotensin-converting enzyme inhibitor (ACEI) or angiotensin receptor blocker (ARB).

There were 144 patients registered with the practice with heart failure – 112 of them were on an ACEI or ARB (78%). She printed off a list of patients on the heart failure register but who were not on an ACEI or ARB and started checking their notes. Five patients had terminal illnesses (two widespread metastatic cancer, one end-stage dementia, one advanced Parkinson's disease and one motor neurone disease). They were valid exceptions. This took the denominator down to 139, and the percentage on an ACEI/ARB to 81%, qualifying for the maximum payment.

Think laterally

Every practice is different but there are many ways in which individual practices have made data collection for QOF purposes easier. The following are examples from practices that we have experience of.

- Give every patient a brief questionnaire, asking height, weight, smoking status and alcohol consumption, to complete in the waiting room while waiting for any appointment and to hand back to the receptionist.

- Consider installing a self-service blood pressure monitor allowing patients to check their own blood pressure in the waiting room. Ensure blood pressures checked in this way are automatically recorded on computer or given in to the receptionist before the patient leaves.
- At the time of the annual influenza vaccination clinics, consider trawling patients expected to attend for those who have defaulted from chronic disease management clinics. Ensure a clinician is present at each flu clinic who can target and perform basic QOF checks on these patients while they are in the surgery.

Link QOF to other practice activities

The QOF is only one element in the running of a practice. QOF activities should not be seen in isolation. Try to link QOF activity into other practice activities to economise on resources. For example, link reviews of medication to prescribing reviews.

DECIDING WHEN ENOUGH IS ENOUGH

With increasing financial pressures on practices, and more competition from other providers, the temptation is to try to achieve every QOF point. However, as QOF points become harder to achieve, practices have to decide for themselves whether chasing every QOF point is cost-efficient.

It is important to find out precisely what achieving the target will entail. If additional work is needed, it is important to look at who will do that work and how much that additional work will cost the practice. If meeting a new target entails extra expense, it is important to weigh up whether that additional expenditure is counterbalanced either by the additional income or other benefits to the practice – for example, in terms of better patient care.

CONCLUSIONS

P4P is still an imperfect approach to improving primary care and should be considered as only one option alongside alternative quality improvement methods. Policymakers in other countries should exercise caution before implementing similar schemes. Consideration should be given to improving different dimensions of quality, including user experience, and equity. Costs should be monitored and balanced against benefits.

The QOF has become a powerful force influencing every aspect of primary care practice in the United Kingdom. QOF achievement is largely decided on the basis of the quality of data collected by a practice. This results in both clinical and administrative challenges for practices if they are to achieve their maximum QOF potential.

REFERENCES

Checkland K, Harrison S (2010) The impact of the Quality and Outcomes Framework on practice organisation and service delivery: summary of evidence from two qualitative studies. *Qual Prim Care.* **18**(12): 139–46.

Doran T, Fullwood C, Kontopantelis E, *et al.* (2008a) Effect of financial incentives on inequalities in the delivery of primary clinical care in England: analysis of clinical activity indicators for the quality and outcomes framework. *Lancet.* **372**(9640): 728–36.

Doran T, Fullwood C, Reeves D, *et al.* (2008b) Exclusion of patients from pay-for-performance targets by English physicians. *N Engl J Med.* **359**(3): 274–84.

Doran T, Kontopantelis E, Valderas JM, *et al.* (2011) Effect of financial incentives on incentivised and non-incentivised clinical activities: longitudinal analysis of data from the UK Quality and Outcomes Framework. *BMJ.* **342**: d3590.

Fleetcroft R, Parekh-Bhurke S, Howe A, *et al.* (2010) The UK pay-for-performance programme in primary care: estimation of population mortality reduction. *Br J Gen Pract.* **60**(578): e345–52.

Gillam S, Siriwardena AN (2010) *The Quality and Outcomes Framework: QOF transforming general practice.* Radcliffe Publishing: Oxford.

Gillam S, Siriwardena N, Steel N (2012) Pay-for-performance in the UK: the impact of the Quality and Outcomes Framework – a systematic review. *Ann Fam Med.* **10**(5): 461–8. Available at: http://annfammed.org/content/10/5/461.full (accessed 22 June 2014).

Health and Social Care Information Centre (2013) *Quality and Outcomes Framework Achievement, prevalence and exceptions data 2012/3.* HSCIS: London. Available at: www. hscic.gov.uk/catalogue/PUB12262/qual-outc-fram-12-13-rep.pdf (accessed 22 June 2014).

Mant J, Hicks N (1995) Detecting differences in quality of care: the sensitivity of measures of process and outcome in treating acute myocardial infarction. *BMJ.* **311**(7008): 793–6.

Marshall M, Harrison S (2005) It's about more than money: financial incentives and internal motivation. *Qual Saf Health Care.* **14**(1): 4–5.

McGregor W, Jabareen H, O'Donnell CA, *et al.* (2008) Impact of the 2004 GMS contract on practice nurses: a qualitative study. *Br J Gen Pract.* **58**(555): 711–19.

Reeves D, Doran T, Valderas JM, *et al.* (2010) How to identify when a performance indicator has run its course. *BMJ.* **340**: c1717.

Roland M (2004) Linking physicians' pay to the quality of care: a major experiment in the United Kingdom. *N Engl J Med.* **351**(14): 1448–54.

Scott A, Sivey P, Ait OD, *et al.* (2011) The effect of financial incentives on the quality of health care provided by primary care physicians. *Cochrane Database Syst Rev.* (9): CD008451.

Shohet C, Yelloly J, Bingham P, *et al.* (2007) The association between the quality of epilepsy management in primary care, general practice population deprivation status and epilepsy-related emergency hospitalisations. *Seizure.* **16**(4): 351–5.

Simon C, Morton A (2010) Getting the most out of the QOF. In: Gillam S, Siriwardena AN (eds). *The Quality and Outcomes Framework: QOF transforming general practice.* Radcliffe Publishing: Oxford. pp. 111–27.

Walker S, Mason AR, Claxton K, *et al.* (2010) Value for money and the Quality and Outcomes Framework in primary care in the UK NHS. *Br J Gen Pract.* **60**(574): 213–20.

Wilkie P (2010) Does the patient always benefit? In: Gillam S, Siriwardena AN (eds). *The Quality and Outcomes Framework: QOF transforming general practice.* Radcliffe Publishing: Oxford. pp. 128–36.

Evaluation and personal development

CHAPTER 10

Evaluating improvement

SUMMARY

- Clinical audit and quality improvement projects can be used to evaluate healthcare initiatives – these methods are covered in Chapters 5 and 7.
- More detailed evaluation of quality improvement interventions requires a variety of methods, ranging from quantitative methods such as randomised controlled trials (RCTs) to quasi-experimental (controlled before-and-after and interrupted time series) and uncontrolled before-and-after studies.
- Qualitative methods are often also used to understand how or why an intervention was successful and which components of a complex or multifaceted intervention were most effective.
- Mixed methods designs such as action research or case study methods are widely used to design and evaluate improvement interventions.

INTRODUCTION

A range of methods have been used to evaluate quality improvement interventions in primary care. These can vary in terms of the rigour of the methods used and their ability to attribute improvement to the intervention being proposed. Clinical audit and quality improvement projects can be used to evaluate improvement initiatives and should be within the scope of practitioners.

More rigorous studies require support from academic teams with expertise in these methods. Studies can range in design from RCTs, where attribution is clearer, to other types of experimental methods, including quasi-experimental designs such as non-randomised control group (sometimes called controlled before-and-after) or interrupted time series methods to uncontrolled before-and-after studies (including clinical audits), where attribution is less certain (*see* Figure 10.1) (Siriwardena 2013).

Improvement interventions are often complex (i.e. multiple rather than single) and pragmatic, so that 'real-world' designs are called for. Improvement often involves a series of interventions including education (of professionals and/or patients), reminders (to professionals and/or patients), audit and feedback or other measures. These vary in content, intensity or timing between different intervention sites so that it is not always clear which components of the 'black box' of the intervention are effective (Siriwardena 2008).

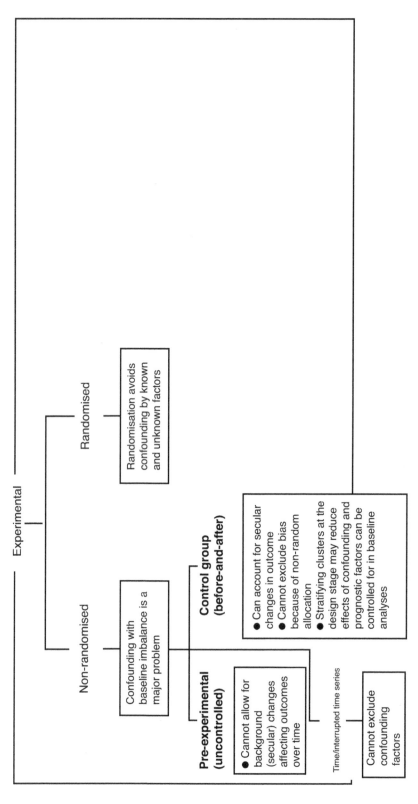

FIGURE 10.1 Experimental studies used to evaluate improvement interventions (adapted from Ukoumunne, *et al.* 1999)

In order to understand how or why an intervention works it is often necessary to use methods such as surveys or qualitative interviews, focus groups, documentary (textual) analysis, observational or ethnographic methods. It may also be necessary to combine quantitative and qualitative methods (e.g. with case study methods), or to work with participants to design the evaluation (e.g. using action research methods). Quality improvement methods themselves can also be used to evaluate improvement, which adds to the complexities of improvement evaluations (Siriwardena 2009).

DESIGNING EVALUATIONS

A starting point for designing a formal evaluation is the logic model based on the specific question the evaluation is trying to answer. Logic models (*see* Chapter 6) can also be used to design improvement interventions by defining the population and problem that the intervention is aimed at, specifying inputs (in terms of resources provided for planning, implementation and evaluation), outputs (in terms of healthcare processes implemented and the population that is actually reached) and longer-term outcomes measured in terms of health and wider benefits or harms, whether intended or incidental and in the short, medium or long term (Siriwardena 2009).

In an evaluation logic model we can add to this by specifying the evidence or data to be collected and the method that will be used to analyse the data. For example, the logic model for an evaluation of a national quality improvement collaborative designed to improve care for acute myocardial infarction and stroke in ambulance services is shown (*see* Figure 10.2) (Siriwardena, *et al.* 2014).

This shows that we collected quantitative data, survey data (pre and post intervention), qualitative data from observations and meetings and analysed these using a mixture of time series, qualitative analysis, pattern matching to link time series and qualitative findings, and comparison of different sites (cross-case synthesis) to develop an explanation of what happened, i.e. why and how improvement came about as a result of the collaborative.

We describe the individual methods used to determine effect sizes of improvement interventions and to understand how or why an intervention was successful or which components of a complex, multifaceted intervention were most effective.

RANDOMISED CONTROLLED TRIALS

Because improvement interventions usually involve education of healthcare staff together with other multiple components, the commonest type of RCT used is the cluster randomised controlled trial (CRCT). CRCTs involve randomisation of practitioners or groups of practitioners (in a practice, organisation or area), rather than individual patients, allocated to an intervention or control group.

CRCTs are used because educational interventions for professionals cannot be switched on and off with different patients – that is, professionals are not able to implement their learning with one patient randomised to the intervention while forgetting what they have learned with another patient allocated to a control group.

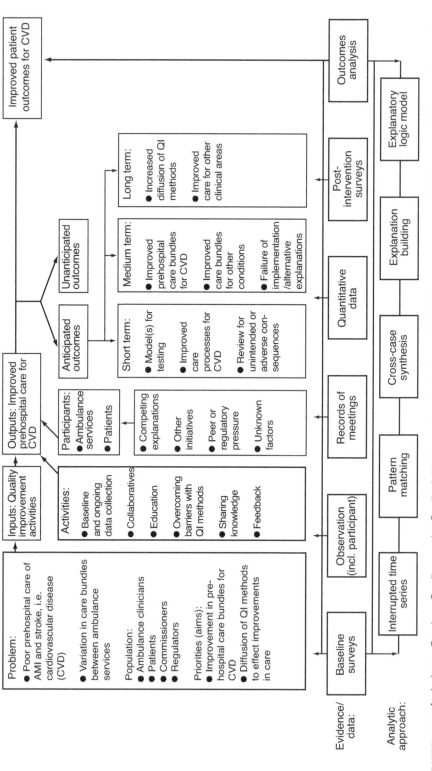

FIGURE 10.2 Ambulance Services Cardiovascular Quality Initiative: evaluation logic model (AMI = acute myocardial infarction; CVD = cardiovascular disease; QI = quality improvement) (Siriwardena, *et al.* 2014)

The unit of analysis in CRCTs can be at the level of the unit of randomisation or at the level of the patient. Although many design flaws of RCTs can also apply to CRCTs (e.g. allocation bias, volunteer bias), there are additional features that should be considered in CRCTs. These include the potential correlation of outcomes between patients in clusters (termed the intra-cluster correlation) that occurs because these patients tend to be more similar to one another than to a randomly selected patient. There is an additional risk of patients in control clusters receiving the intervention. This can occur because professionals in the intervention arm move to the control cluster (i.e. switch organisations or locations) or because those in the control arm learn about the intervention from colleagues in the intervention arm, an occurrence that is termed 'contamination'.

An example of a CRCT of an improvement intervention is outlined in Box 10.1. In this example both the unit of randomisation and analysis was the practice.

BOX 10.1 Case study – cluster randomised controlled trial of an educational outreach visit to improve influenza and pneumococcal immunisation rates in primary care

Improvement in the delivery of influenza and pneumococcal vaccinations to high-risk groups is an important aspect of preventive care delivered by primary healthcare teams. We aimed to investigate the effect of an educational outreach intervention to primary healthcare teams on influenza and pneumococcal vaccination uptake in high-risk patients.

We used a CRCT design. The trial involved 30 general practices in the Trent region of the United Kingdom. Fifteen practices were randomised to the intervention and 15 to the control group after stratifying for baseline vaccination rate. All intervention practices were offered and received an educational outreach visit to primary healthcare teams, in addition to audit and feedback directed at improving influenza and pneumococcal vaccination rates in high-risk groups. Control practices received audit and feedback alone. We measured influenza and pneumococcal vaccination rates in high-risk groups in all practices. Primary outcomes were improvements in vaccination rates in patients aged 65 years and over, and in patients with coronary heart disease (CHD), diabetes and a history of splenectomy.

Improvements in pneumococcal vaccination rates in the intervention practices were significantly greater than with controls in patients with CHD (14.8% versus 6.5%; risk ratio [RR] 1.23; 95% confidence interval [CI] 1.13–1.34) and diabetes (15.5% versus 6.8%; RR 1.18; 95% CI 1.08–1.29) but not splenectomy (6.5% versus 4.7%; RR 0.96; 95% CI 0.65–1.42). Improvements for influenza vaccination were also usually greater in intervention practices but did not reach statistical significance. The increases for influenza vaccination in intervention versus control practices were for CHD (18.1% versus 13.1%; RR 1.06; 95% CI 0.99–1.12), diabetes (15.5% versus 12.0%; RR 1.07; 95% CI 0.99–1.16), splenectomy (16.1% versus 2.9%; RR 1.22; 95% CI 0.78–1.93), and those over 65 years of age (20.7% versus 25.4%; RR 0.99; 95% CI 0.96–1.02).

We found that practices where primary care teams received an educational outreach visit demonstrated a significantly greater improvement in uptake in high-risk groups for pneumococcal but not influenza vaccine.

(Siriwardena, *et al.* 2002)

BEFORE-AND-AFTER STUDIES

Single-group before-and-after (or pre-post-intervention) studies without a control group, sometimes termed pre-experimental studies, are often used in improvement studies. An example is outlined in Box 10.2.

BOX 10.2 Case study – before-and-after study evaluating improvement in influenza and pneumococcal vaccination uptake in high-risk groups in Lincolnshire

The delivery of influenza and pneumococcal vaccine to high-risk groups is an important preventive care responsibility for primary care.

We used a two-stage multipractice audit of influenza and pneumococcal vaccination rates in high-risk groups before and after graphical anonymised feedback and written advice on improving vaccination rates.

Twenty-two out of 105 Lincolnshire practices volunteered to participate. The study period for the baseline data collection was September–December 1998 and re-evaluation took place in January–February 2000 after the next annual influenza vaccination programme. Key measures for improvement were influenza and pneumococcal vaccination rates in high-risk groups, specifically in patients with CHD, diabetes and post splenectomy.

A combination of strategies for change were used including dissemination of guidelines, advice on setting up disease and vaccine registers, organisational strategies for improving vaccination rates such as call and recall systems and benchmarking of performance.

For practices participating in both phases of the audit cycle, mean annual influenza vaccination uptake increased by 10.8% (95% CI 5.3–16.1; $p = 0.001$) to 74.4% in CHD patients, by 8.6% (95% CI 1.5–15.7; $p = 0.02$) to 70.6% in patients with diabetes, and by 17.3% (95% CI 4.8–29.8; $p = 0.01$) in patients post splenectomy. Mean pneumococcal vaccination rates improved by 27.5% (95% CI 12.6–42.3; $p = 0.002$) to 58.6% in CHD patients, by 28.8% (95% CI 17.2–40.3; $p < 0.001$) to 64.0% in patients with diabetes, and by 15.9% (95% CI 1.8–30.1; $p = 0.03$) in post-splenectomy patients. These improvements occurred prior to the current national programme for influenza vaccination of patients over 65 years of age.

Improvements in influenza and pneumococcal vaccination uptake occurred in patients with CHD, diabetes and post splenectomy at re-evaluation. Practices were able to achieve and exceed national targets for influenza immunisation of high-risk groups. Quality of care improved through organisational change, audit and feedback with benchmarking of performance.

(Siriwardena, *et al.* 2003)

Pre-experimental designs suffer from significant and often irremediable flaws. It may be impossible to determine whether an improvement or other change in outcome is due to the intervention itself or to a confounding or alternative explanation, such as an external factor or a natural change over time, the latter referred to as a secular trend. Outcomes may also be altered because of the participants changing their behaviour as a result of being observed (the Hawthorne effect) or due to regression to the mean, where outlying variables tend to move towards mean values. However, they may be useful for developing an improvement intervention prior to more rigorous testing.

QUASI-EXPERIMENTAL STUDIES

Quasi-experimental trials are more robust than pre-experimental studies but less so than RCTs. There are two main types of quasi-experimental study: the non-randomised controlled before-and-after study and the (interrupted) time series study. In the controlled before-and-after design an intervention is administered to a study group and compared with a control group who continue as usual. An example is outlined in Box 10.3. Confounding may be due to external influences on outcomes occurring between the pre-intervention and post-intervention phases. Potential sources of bias include selection bias, from non-random selection of intervention and control groups or areas, leading to baseline imbalance in outcomes of other differences between the two groups. Regression to the mean and differences in secular trends between groups may also occur in such studies.

BOX 10.3 Case study – an evaluation of an educational intervention to reduce inappropriate cannulation and improve cannulation technique by paramedics

Intravenous cannulation enables administration of fluids or drugs by paramedics in the prehospital setting. Inappropriate use and poor technique carry risks for patients, including pain and infection. We aimed to investigate the effect of an educational intervention designed to reduce the rate of inappropriate cannulation and to improve cannulation technique.

We used a non-randomised control group design, comparing two counties in the East Midlands of the United Kingdom as intervention and control areas. The educational intervention was based on Joint Royal Colleges Ambulance Liaison Committee guidance and delivered to paramedic team leaders who cascaded it to their teams. We analysed rates of inappropriate cannulation before and after the intervention using routine clinical data. We also assessed overall cannulation rates before and after the intervention. A sample of paramedics was assessed post intervention on cannulation technique with a 'model' arm using a predesigned checklist.

There was a non-significant reduction in inappropriate (no intravenous fluids or drugs given) cannulation rates in the intervention area (from 1.0% to 0%) compared with the control area (from 2.5% to 2.6%). There was a significant ($p < 0.001$) reduction in cannulation rates in the intervention area (from 9.1% to 6.5%; odds ratio [OR] 0.7, 95% CI 0.48–1.03) compared with an increase in the control area (from 13.8% to 19.1%; OR 1.47, 95% CI 1.15–1.90), a significant difference ($p < 0.001$). Paramedics in the intervention area were significantly more likely to use correct handwashing techniques post intervention (74.5% versus 14.9%; $p < 0.001$).

The educational intervention was effective in bringing about changes leading to enhanced quality and safety in some aspects of prehospital cannulation.

(Siriwardena, *et al.* 2009)

The interrupted time series design looks at data for the outcome of interest for a period of time before, during and after the intervention and therefore takes secular trends before the intervention into account. However, this design can be affected by loss to follow-up (or attrition), Hawthorne effects or contamination. An example is outlined in Box 10.4.

BOX 10.4 Case study – investigation of the effect of a countywide protected learning time scheme on prescribing rates of ramipril using an interrupted time series design

Protected learning time (PLT) schemes were set up in primary care across the United Kingdom with little published evidence of their effectiveness.

We wished to investigate the effect of a PLT intervention for general practice in Lincolnshire, in the United Kingdom, to increase prescribing of ramipril for the prevention of adverse cardiovascular outcomes.

We used a quasi-experimental, interrupted time series design. We analysed prescribing data 1 year before and after the education investigating change in rate of increase of prescribing of ramipril, whether change in prescribing was related to postulated explanatory variables and to determine intervention costs.

The primary outcome was the rate of change of ramipril (10 mg) prescription items 12 months after compared with before the educational intervention. Secondary outcomes included cost. Ramipril prescribing at therapeutic dosage increased significantly (OR 1.50; 95% CI 1.07–1.93) following education by 52 345 items (31 132 items at 10 mg) at a cost of £292k–£460k, depending on the drug formulation. This occurred despite a background of secular change.

Most practices were represented by general practitioners (GPs), nurses or both during the education. Single-handed GPs were less likely to attend. Practices showed considerable variation in response to the educational intervention. The only predictor of whether practices increased in prescribing rate after the education was whether a practice nurse had undertaken specific diabetes training. Total list size, dispensing, training or single-handed status and GP attendance did not predict a change in prescribing.

We concluded that PLT schemes can contribute to beneficial changes in prescribing across a large geographical area.

(Siriwardena, *et al.* 2006)

QUALITATIVE METHODS

Although experimental methods can show the extent of any change resulting from an improvement initiative, they cannot explain why or how the change occurred without using qualitative methods. Qualitative methods can take the form of interviews (of patients or practitioners or both), focus groups and observations including ethnographic methods and these can provide in-depth information about how and why an improvement intervention might be working (*see* Box 10.5).

BOX 10.5 Case study – qualitative interview study of practitioners exploring drivers for change in primary care of diabetes following a protected learning time educational event

A number of PLT schemes have been set up in primary care across the United Kingdom but there has been little published evidence of their impact on processes of care. We undertook a qualitative study to investigate the perceptions of practitioners involved in a specific educational intervention in diabetes as part of a PLT scheme for primary healthcare teams, relating to changing processes of diabetes care in general practice.

We undertook semi-structured interviews of key informants from a sample of practices stratified according to the extent they had changed behaviour in prescribing of ramipril and diabetes care more generally, following a specific educational intervention in Lincolnshire, in the United Kingdom. Interviews sought information on facilitators and barriers to change in organisational behaviour for the care of diabetes.

An inter-professional PLT scheme event was perceived by some but not all participants as bringing about changes in processes for diabetes care. Participants cited examples of change introduced partly as a result of the educational session. This included using ACE inhibitors as first line for patients with diabetes who developed hypertension, increased use of aspirin, switching patients to glitazones, and conversion to insulin either directly or by referral to secondary care. Other reported factors for change, unrelated to the educational intervention, included financially driven performance targets, research evidence and national guidance.

Facilitators for change linked to the educational session were peer support and team-working supported by audit and comparative feedback.

A protected learning time scheme, using inter-professional learning, local opinion leaders and early implementers as change agents influenced changes in systems of diabetes care in selected practices but also affected how other confounding factors brought about change.

(Siriwardena, *et al.* 2008)

ACTION RESEARCH, CASE STUDY AND MIXED METHODS

Evaluations of improvement often involve mixed methods, combining quantitative and qualitative methods to determine both the effect size and determinants of an improvement intervention. Action research studies involve participants to a greater or lesser extent in the conception, design and evaluation of an intervention designed to bring about change; they evaluate the effects of an improvement intervention.

Case study methods may be based on a single case or multiple cases (Yin 2003). They combine methods to develop an explanatory model for why an intervention might work in some cases and not in others. For example, in the Ambulance Services Cardiovascular Quality Initiative (*see* Figure 10.2 and Box 10.6) we combined interrupted time series and multiple case study methods, matching the patterns of change in ambulance services with a detailed analysis of changes within each service to develop an explanation of what led to differences in improvement.

BOX 10.6 Case study – effect of a national quality improvement collaborative on prehospital care for acute myocardial infarction and stroke in England

Previous studies have shown wide variations in prehospital ambulance care for acute myocardial infarction (AMI) and stroke. We aimed to evaluate the effectiveness of implementing a quality improvement collaborative (QIC) for improving ambulance care for AMI and stroke.

We used an interrupted time series design to investigate the effect of a national QIC on change in delivery of care bundles for AMI (aspirin, glyceryl trinitrate, pain assessment and analgesia) and stroke (face-arm-speech test, blood pressure and blood glucose recording) in all English ambulance services between January 2010 and February 2012. Key strategies for change included local quality improvement (QI) teams in each ambulance service, supported by a national coordinating expert group that conducted workshops educating staff in QI methods to improve AMI and stroke care. Expertise and ideas were shared between QI teams who met together at three national workshops, between QI leads through monthly teleconferences and between the expert group and participants. Feedback was provided to services using annotated control charts.

We analysed change over time using logistic regression with three predictor variables: time, gender and age. There were statistically significant improvements in care bundles in nine (of 12) participating trusts for AMI (OR 1.04; 95% CI 1.04–1.04), nine for stroke (OR 1.06; 95% CI 1.05–1.07), 11 for either AMI or stroke, and seven for both conditions. Overall care bundle performance for AMI increased in England from 43% to 79% and for stroke from 83% to 96%. Successful services all introduced provider prompts and individualised or team feedback. Other determinants of success included engagement with front-line clinicians, feedback using annotated control charts, expert support, and shared learning between participants and organisations.

The QIC led to significant improvements in ambulance care for AMI and stroke in England. The use of care bundles as measures, clinical engagement, application of QI methods, provider prompts, individualised feedback and opportunities for learning and interaction within and across organisations helped the collaborative to achieve its aims.

(Siriwardena, *et al.* 2014)

CONCLUSION

Evaluating quality improvement interventions requires a variety of methods. These range from quantitative methods such as RCTs, to quasi-experimental (controlled before-and-after and interrupted time series) and uncontrolled before-and-after studies to determine whether improvement interventions have had an effect. Qualitative methods are often also used to understand how or why an intervention was successful and which components of a complex or multifaceted intervention were most effective. Finally, mixed methods designs such as action research or case study methods are widely used to design and evaluate improvement interventions.

REFERENCES

Siriwardena AN (2013) Experimental methods in health research. In: Saks M, Allsop J (eds). *Researching health: qualitative, quantitative and mixed methods.* Sage: London. pp. 263–79.

Siriwardena AN (2009) Using quality improvement methods for evaluating health care. *Qual Prim Care.* **17**(3): 155–9.

Siriwardena AN (2008) The exceptional potential for quality improvement methods in the design and modelling of complex interventions. *Qual Prim Care.* **16**(6): 387–9.

Siriwardena AN, Fairchild P, Gibson S, *et al.* (2006) Investigation of the effect of a county-wide protected learning time scheme on prescribing rates of ramipril: interrupted time series study. *Fam Pract.* Epub Oct 18.

Siriwardena AN, Rashid A, Johnson M, *et al.* (2003) Improving influenza and pneumococcal vaccination uptake in high-risk groups in Lincolnshire: a quality improvement report from a large rural county. *Qual Prim Care.* **11**: 19–28.

Siriwardena AN, Iqbal M, Banerjee S, *et al.* (2009) An evaluation of an educational intervention to reduce inappropriate cannulation and improve cannulation technique by paramedics. *Emerg Med J.* **26**(11): 831–6.

Siriwardena AN, Middlemass JB, Ward K, *et al.* (2008) Drivers for change in primary care of diabetes following a protected learning time educational event: interview study of practitioners. *BMC Med Educ.* **8**: 4.

Siriwardena AN, Rashid A, Johnson MR, *et al.* (2002) Cluster randomised controlled trial of an educational outreach visit to improve influenza and pneumococcal immunisation rates in primary care. *Br J Gen Pract.* **52**(482): 735–40.

Siriwardena AN, Shaw D, Essam N, *et al.* (2014) The effect of a national quality improvement collaborative on prehospital care for acute myocardial infarction and stroke in England. *Implement Sci.* **9**: 17.

Ukoumunne OC, Gulliford MC, Chinn S, *et al.* (1999) Methods for evaluating area-wide and organisation-based interventions in health and healthcare: a systematic review. *Health Technol Assess.* **3**(5): iii-92.

Yin RK (2003) *Case study research: design and methods.* Sage: Thousand Oaks, CA.

CHAPTER 11

Evidence-based healthcare

SUMMARY

- Sound evidence underpins the translation of knowledge for improvement in healthcare practice and patient outcomes.
- Evidence-based practice integrates the individual practitioner's experience, patient preferences and the best available research information.
- Incorporating the best available research evidence in decision-making involves five steps: (1) *asking* answerable questions, (2) *accessing* the best information, (3) *appraising* the information for validity and relevance, (4) *applying* the information to care of patients and populations and (5) *evaluating* the impact for evidence of change and expected outcomes.
- Major barriers to implementing evidence-based practice include the impression among practitioners that their professional freedom is being constrained, lack of appropriate training and resource constraints.
- Financial incentives, guidance and regulation are increasingly being used to encourage evidence-based practice but should not override the interests of individual patients.

INTRODUCTION

For QI initiatives to be effective, they should be based on sound evidence. However, there are two main considerations relating to this evidence base. First, the intervention or interventions that the QI initiative seeks to implement should have evidence of benefit: they should lead to improvements in patient outcomes that are, ideally, both clinically important and cost-effective. The evidence that translates basic research to its clinical application through new health technologies (either products or approaches) has been termed the 'first translational gap'.

Second, QI initiatives should be based on sound evidence of what works to implement these products or approaches. This is the 'second translational gap' that forms the basis of quality improvement and implementation science (Cooksey 2006). We now consider evidence-based healthcare (EBHC) in the context of both these translational gaps.

WHAT IS EVIDENCE-BASED HEALTHCARE?

How much of what health and other professionals do is based soundly in science? Answers to the question 'Is our practice evidence based?' depend on what we mean by practice and what we mean by evidence. This varies from discipline to discipline. A study in general practice found that around 31% of therapeutic clinical decisions were based on evidence from randomised controlled trials (RCTs), while 51% were based on convincing non-experimental evidence (Gill, *et al.* 1996).

Sackett, *et al.* (2007) defined evidence-based medicine as

> the conscientious, explicit, and judicious use of current best evidence in making decisions about the care of individual patients . . . integrating individual clinical expertise with the best available external clinical evidence from systematic research.

The expansion of evidence-based medicine has been a major influence on clinical practice over the last 20 years. The demands of purchasers of healthcare, keen to optimise value for money, have been one driver; a growing awareness among health professionals and their patients of medicine's potential to cause harm has been another. In this chapter we examine the nature of what is nowadays more broadly referred to as evidence-based healthcare, or EBHC, in the context of QI and we will discuss its strengths and limitations.

THE TOOLS NECESSARY FOR EVIDENCE-BASED HEALTHCARE

The tools needed to practise in an evidence-based way are common across healthcare disciplines. Doctors, nurses and allied health professionals all need the skills to ensure that the work they do – whether with individual clients or patients, or in the development of policies for quality improvement – is based on sound knowledge of what is likely to work.

Of the following five essential steps, the first is probably the most important:
1 convert information needs into answerable questions (i.e. by asking a focused question)
2 track down the best available evidence
3 appraise evidence critically
4 change practice in the light of evidence
5 evaluate your performance.

STEP 1: ASKING A FOCUSED QUESTION

Before seeking the best evidence, you need to convert your information needs into a tightly focused question. For example, it is not enough to ask: 'Are antibiotics effective for otitis media?' We need to convert this into an answerable question: 'Do antibiotics reduce the duration of symptoms when prescribed to children with otitis media?'

The PICO approach can be used as a framework to focus a question by considering the necessary elements. It contains four components:
1 Patient or the population (children under 5 years)
2 Intervention (antibiotics)
3 Comparison intervention (placebo)
4 Outcome (duration of specific symptoms, e.g. pain, or rate of complications).

Question
Form a focused clinical question using the PICO format to find the evidence for the effectiveness of smoking-cessation interventions in adult smokers who have had a heart attack.

Answer
P   Adult smokers who have had a heart attack.
I   Providing smoking cessation intervention.
C   Providing usual care.
O   Mortality and quit rates.

This gives us the question, 'In smokers who have had a heart attack, does a smoking-cessation intervention in comparison with usual care reduce mortality and improve quit rate?' (Korenstein and McGinn 2008).

STEP 2: TRACKING DOWN THE EVIDENCE

The second step in the practice of EBHC is to track down the best evidence. Doctors and nurses often assess outcomes in terms of surrogate pathological end points rather than commonplace changes in quality of life or the ability to perform routine activities ('the operation was a success but the patient died').

Traditionally, doctors making decisions about what works have attached much weight to personal experience or the views of respected colleagues. Over time, knowledge of up-to-date care diminishes, so there is a constant need for the latest evidence and simple ways to access and use it (Choudhry, *et al.* 2005; Ramsey, *et al.* 1991). A study of North American physicians has shown that up-to-date clinical information is needed twice for every three patients seen, but they only receive 30% of this because of lack of time, dated textbooks and disorganised journals (Covell, *et al.* 1985).

Rather than relying on colleagues or textbooks, EBHC encourages the use of research evidence in a systematic way. Once a question has been formulated, the research base is then searched to find articles of relevance.

So what counts as evidence? Care needs to be taken in relying on published articles. Many reviews reflect the prejudices of their authors and are anything but systematic. Even mainstream journals tend to accept papers yielding positive rather than negative findings – for example, in assessing treatments, so-called 'publication bias' (Easterbrook, *et al.* 1991; Dickersin 1990). Most books date rapidly. Hence the prominence nowadays accorded to properly conducted systematic reviews, which are placed at the top of a 'hierarchy' of evidence. A widely used ranking of the strength of evidence is shown in Table 11.1 (Scottish Intercollegiate Guidelines Network 2014).

Table 11.1 reminds us of the three main types of epidemiological study design: (1) descriptive, (2) observational and (3) interventional. When searching for evidence we should look for the highest level suitable to our question. A question relating to the effectiveness of an intervention will most appropriately be answered by a RCT or a systematic review of RCTs.

The RCT is widely regarded as the 'gold standard' method for determining effectiveness, as robust randomisation ensures that study and control groups

TABLE 11.1 Levels of evidence for clinical practice guidelines (Scottish Intercollegiate Guideline Network)

Level	Source of evidence
1++	High-quality meta-analyses, systematic reviews of RCTs, or RCTs with a very low risk of bias
1+	Well-conducted meta-analyses, systematic reviews or RCTs with a low risk of bias
1–	Meta-analyses, systematic reviews or RCTs with a high risk of bias
2++	High-quality systematic reviews of case–control or cohort studies; high-quality case–control or cohort studies with a very low risk of confounding or bias and a high probability that the relationship is causal
2+	Well-conducted case–control or cohort studies with a low risk of confounding or bias and a moderate probability that the relationship is causal
2–	Case–control or cohort studies with a high risk of confounding or bias and a significant risk that the relationship is not causal
3	Non-analytic studies (e.g. case reports, case series)
4	Expert opinion

RCT = randomised controlled trial

differ only in terms of their exposure to the factor under study; the observed results are due only to the intervention and not to alternative explanations (so-called confounding variables). The Scottish Intercollegiate Guidelines Network takes into account the potential biases in its hierarchy of evidence. We can find answers to questions about the possible causes of a disease from associations generated by case–control or cohort studies.

However, questions beginning 'Why?' or 'How?' are often not answered by these kinds of study. What factors, after all, go to make a 'good nurse' or a 'good public health practitioner' and how easily are they measured? It is not possible to answer the question, 'Why do women refuse an offer of breast screening?' with any of the study types mentioned so far. Another example would be: 'How do medicines get prescribed inappropriately in older patients?' In these cases one looks for a qualitative study. Qualitative studies use methods such as interviews, diaries and direct observation to provide detailed information to describe the experiences of participants. Qualitative data are then analysed rigorously to lead to conclusions about why or how something might have occurred (Pope and Mays 2006). Detailed coverage of qualitative methodology is beyond the scope of this chapter, but it is important to remember that not every question can be answered using the classical hierarchy outlined here. Qualitative methods can generate a wealth of knowledge to contextualise many of the decisions health professionals must make.

Question
Consider the questions below. What studies would be most appropriately conducted to answer them: RCT, cohort, case–control, cross-sectional, qualitative?
a   For what conditions do patients call their GP out-of-hours?
b   What are the barriers to handwashing in healthcare settings?

c   Does paternal exposure to ionising radiation before conception cause childhood leukaemia?

d   What is the most sensitive and specific method of screening for genital chlamydial infection in women attending general practice?

e   Does laparoscopic cholecystectomy cause less morbidity and a swifter return to work than a small-incision cholecystectomy?

f   Do clinicians change their practice as a result of education?

g   For a given patient with asthma, does beclometasone give better symptomatic control than fluticasone?

h   How do patients and carers view the service provided by a mental health team?

i   How does smoking cessation affect the risk of stroke in middle-aged men?

Answer

a   Cross-sectional study
b   Qualitative study
c   Case–control study
d   Cross-sectional study
e   RCT
f   Cohort study
g   RCT
h   Qualitative study
i   Cohort study

There are various primary and secondary sources of evidence. Primary sources are the thousands of original papers published every year in research journals. However, to deal with the vast amount of information available, more and more people now turn to secondary sources of evidence. The single most important source of systematic reviews is the Cochrane Database (www. cochrane.org). The Cochrane Collaboration (as mentioned in the Introduction, named after Archie Cochrane, an early pioneer of evidence-based medicine) is an international endeavour to summarise high-quality evidence in all fields of medical practice. It has slowly transformed many areas of clinical practice.

It is important to have basic skills in searching the literature, although the help of expert librarians may be needed. Research papers are catalogued in a variety of databases searchable on the Internet. For many medical or public health queries the database MEDLINE is a good starting place. Other databases are available for specialist queries, such as those in the fields of mental health and nursing. Using the PICO format here is helpful, as it can be used to generate search terms with which to query the databases. Databases may have tools to support the user in this such as the 'Clinical Queries' tool in PubMed, which is a US National Library of Medicine's service to search the biomedical research literature.

We can use our example question from earlier to demonstrate how a search might work. Our focused question was, 'In smokers who have had a heart attack, does a smoking-cessation intervention in comparison with usual care reduce mortality and improve quit rate?'

Question
What study type would be appropriate for answering this question?

Answer
RCTs are possible, where smokers who have had a heart attack are randomised to receive smoking-cessation intervention or usual care, to give a measure of the relative effectiveness of smoking-cessation intervention.

Question
Using the PICO format, list the key words we need to use to search databases through a search function such as PubMed's Clinical Queries.

Answer
Smokers, heart attack, cessation, counselling, mortality. In Clinical Queries, as we select an option to indicate our interest is in therapy (i.e. intervention studies) the term 'randomised controlled trial' is automatically added to the key words. In other search systems or databases this may need to be added manually.

The journal articles found using this strategy are as follows.
- NA Rigotti, AN Thorndike, S Regan, *et al.* (2006) Bupropion for smokers hospitalised with acute cardiovascular disease. *Am J Med.* **119**(12): 1080–7.
- EA Dornelas, RA Sampson, JF Gray, *et al.* (2000) A randomised controlled trial of smoking cessation counseling after myocardial infarction. *Prev Med.* **30**(4): 261–8.
- Wilson K, Hettle R, Marbaix S, *et al.* (2012) An economic evaluation based on a randomized placebo-controlled trial of varenicline in smokers with cardiovascular disease: results for Belgium, Spain, Portugal, and Italy. *Eur J Prev Cardiol.* **19**(5): 1173–83.

Question
Look at these results. Are these articles relevant?

Answer
Yes – bupropion is used to help smokers quit their habit. The second study is an RCT testing the effectiveness of smoking cessation in patients who have had a myocardial infarction (heart attack).

In our search for evidence it should be remembered that not every piece of information that might help us answer our question may have been published. There may be studies in progress that could inform our action; negative studies, which could help tell us what *not* to do, may not have made it as far as a publication; many pharmaceutical companies have unpublished information; conference reports might provide helpful information. As we move down the hierarchy it becomes more difficult to find this kind of evidence (called 'grey' literature) from readily available sources but some databases and repositories are available. This is a good time to seek the help of an expert librarian!

STEP 3: APPRAISING THE EVIDENCE

To determine whether we should act on the results of the studies found in the search we must be able to appraise critically a range of study types. An understanding of some basic epidemiological concepts is needed to understand the methods used and the results presented. We are looking to decide whether the results are valid enough to change our practice. In order to do this we ask a series of questions about the study, including:

- Did the researchers ask a clearly focused question and carry out the right sort of study to answer it?
- Were the study methods robust?
- Do the conclusions made match the results of the study? (Might the results have been due to chance? Were they 'big' enough to make a real difference?)
- Can we use these results in our practice?

There are standard checklists available to support systematic appraisal of different types of study designs. We can use these to help determine how valid the findings of the study are, and whether the findings can be generalised to our own population.

Table 11.2 shows a checklist for appraising an RCT, the most appropriate primary design to generate evidence of effective interventions. This checklist is taken from the Critical Appraisal Skills Programme in Oxford (CASP 2014).

TABLE 11.2 Critical Appraisal Skills Programme critical appraisal tool for randomised controlled trials

A	Are the results of the study valid?	
	Screening questions	
1	Did the review ask a clearly focused question?	Yes / Can't tell / No
	Hint – consider if the question is 'focused' in terms of: • the population studied • the intervention given or exposure • the comparator given • the outcomes considered	
2	Was the assignment of patients to treatments randomised?	Yes / Can't tell / No
	Hint – consider: • How was this carried out? • Was the allocation sequence concealed from researchers and patients?	
3	Were all the patients who entered the trial properly accounted for at its conclusion?	Yes / Can't tell / No
	Hint – consider: • Was the trial stopped early? • Were patients analysed in the groups to which they were randomised?	
	Is it worth continuing?	

Detailed questions

4   Were patients, health workers and study personnel 'blind' to treatment?   Yes / Can't tell / No

Hint – think about:
- patients?
- health workers?
- study personnel?

5   Were the groups similar at the start of the trial?   Yes / Can't tell / No

Hint – look at:
- other factors that might affect the outcome, such as age, sex, social class

6   Aside from the experimental intervention were the groups considered equally?   Yes / Can't tell / No

B   What are the results?

7   How large was the treatment effect?

Hint – consider:
- What outcomes were measured?
- Is the primary outcome clearly specified?
- What results were found for each outcome?

8   How precise was the estimate of the treatment effect?

Hint – consider:
- What are the confidence limits?

C   Will the results help locally?

9   Can the results be applied in your context (or to the local population)?   Yes / Can't tell / No

Hint – consider:
- Even if this is not addressed by the review, what do you think?

10   Were all clinically important outcomes considered?   Yes / Can't tell / No

Hint – consider:
- Is there other information you would have liked to have seen?
- Does this affect the decision?

11   Are the benefits worth the harms and costs?   Yes / Can't tell / No

Hint – consider:
- Even if this is not addressed by the review, what do you think?

It is important to be able to critically analyse the results of all study types but, as the volume of scientific literature increases, it is perhaps more important to be able to use systematic reviews effectively to guide practice. It has been estimated that a general physician needs to read for 119 hours a week to keep up to date; medical students are alleged to spend 1–2 hours reading clinical material per week – and that is more than the doctors who teach them (Sackett 2000). Also, a single study of insufficient sample size or of otherwise poor quality may yield misleading results. The right answer to a specific question is more likely to come from a systematic review. This is a review of all the literature on a particular topic, which has been methodically identified, appraised and presented.

The statistical combination of all the results from included studies to provide a summary estimate or definitive result is called meta-analysis.

STEP 4: CHANGING PRACTICE IN THE LIGHT OF EVIDENCE

Following through on the results of your appraisal of new evidence – implementation – is arguably the most difficult of the five steps. Some change can be self-initiated; other circumstances require change in those around you. The implementation of effective interventions often requires change in others. The management of people and an understanding of how they will react to change are invaluable. Implementation strategies may be classified according to the target of the intervention (e.g. patients, providers or systems), the type of intervention (e.g. education, reminders, feedback), or the social theory (e.g. social influence, marketing) that underpins the intervention. The evidence for different types of intervention varies (*see* Box 11.1).

BOX 11.1 Evidence of effectiveness of interventions to change professional behaviour

There is good evidence to support the following.
- **Multifaceted interventions.** By targeting different barriers to change, these are more likely to be effective than single interventions.
- **Educational outreach.** This is generally effective in changing prescribing behaviour in North American settings. Ongoing trials will provide rigorous evidence about the effectiveness of this approach in UK settings.
- **Reminder systems.** These are generally effective for a range of behaviours.

There are mixed effects in the following.
- **Audit and feedback.** These need to be used selectively.
- **Opinion leaders.** These need to be used selectively.

There is little evidence to support the following.
- **Passive dissemination of guidelines.** However, there is some evidence to support use of guidelines if tailored to local needs and associated with reminders.

(NHS Centre for Reviews and Dissemination 1999)

Theoretical models of change and evidence can help us to determine how to implement change. For example, the three main contributors to change are (1) the evidence that underlies the change, (2) the interventions (or facilitators) used to bring about improvement and (3) the context for transformation. The context includes the change agents or various individuals and organisations involved in producing change, including the patient, the provider (healthcare professional), the healthcare team and the various other supporting organisations involved. Quality improvement and implementation efforts will need to embrace this complexity (Siriwardena 2005).

There is no 'magic bullet' (Oxman, *et al.* 1995). Most interventions are effective under some circumstances; none is effective under all circumstances. A diagnostic analysis of the individual and the context must be performed before selecting a method for altering individual practitioner behaviour. Interventions based on assessment of potential barriers are more likely to be effective (Baker, *et al.* 2010).

STEP 5: EVALUATING THE EFFECTS OF CHANGES IN PRACTICE

Commonly, this step will involve a quality improvement project or clinical audit based on an understanding of the processes involved and a framework for improvement. Depending on how frequently the intervention or activity under scrutiny is performed, a review of practice can be undertaken throughout the change using statistical process control methods or before and after the change using a clinical audit.

More robust methods such as RCTs and quasi-experimental (controlled before-and-after and interrupted time series) studies are sometimes used to determine the extent of an improvement; qualitative methods can be used to understand how or why an intervention was successful; and mixed methods, such as action research or case study methods, can be used to do both.

Question
If we go back to the example of use of antibiotics and otitis media from Step 1, how would we know that your practice had changed if we found yourself to be overusing them?

Answer
There are various ways of ascertaining whether practice has changed. You could conduct an audit of the records of all children with a recent diagnosis of otitis media, examine antibiotic prescribing rates before and after introducing the new guidance, survey or interview staff to explore familiarity with the evidence and reasons for their current prescribing practice.

LIMITATIONS TO EVIDENCE-BASED HEALTHCARE

Evidence is only one influence on our practice. Education alone may not change deeply ingrained habits (e.g. patterns of prescribing). Knowledge does not necessarily change practice. This is true for practitioners and patients or the public. An example is the continued use by patients of complementary therapies that professionals consider to be ineffective (Ernst 2002).

Hence we need to consider employing other mechanisms to stimulate change and improvement. These include regulation (*see* Chapter 3) and commissioning (*see* Chapter 4). Commissioning or purchasing can also include financial incentives, which are used to promote interventions known to be effective (e.g. target payments to increase immunisation uptake). In the National Health Service, the Quality and Outcomes Framework system of pay-for-performance was introduced in 2004 to improve the quality of clinical care and promote evidence-based practice (Gillam and Siriwardena 2010), but the evidence for its effectiveness is mixed (*see* Chapter 9) (Gillam, *et al.* 2012).

The most strident criticisms of EBHC have come from those physicians who resent intrusions into their clinical freedom. The use of evidence-based protocols has been demeaned as 'cookbook medicine' (Charlton and Miles 1998). Those who argue that a rigid fixation on RCTs risks ignoring important qualitative sources of evidence mount a more powerful philosophical argument (Popay and Williams 1998).

In addition, there may be times when high-quality evidence simply does not exist. This should not prevent action! The lack of RCTs does not mean an intervention is ineffective, it means that there is no evidence that it is effective, a clear distinction. In these cases, one has to use the best evidence available. When no research evidence exists there is nothing wrong with asking colleagues for their opinions; the practice of EBHC simply means we should at least carry out the search.

CONCLUSION

The terms 'evidence-based medicine' and 'evidence-based healthcare' were developed to encourage practitioners and patients to pay due respect – no more, no less – to current evidence in making decisions. Some 'statistically significant' evidence is clinically insignificant in practice. Evidence should enhance healthcare decision-making, not rigidly dictate it (Greenhalgh, *et al.* 2014). Commercial and managerial interests reflected in protocol-driven care must not be allowed to override shared decision-making in the context of a professional relationship between the clinician and the patient.

FURTHER READING

➡ Greenhalgh T (2010) *How to read a paper: the basics of evidence-based medicine.* Wiley-Blackwell: Chichester, West Sussex.

REFERENCES

Baker R, Camosso-Stefinovic J, Gillies C, *et al.* (2010) Tailored interventions to overcome identified barriers to change: effects on professional practice and health care outcomes. *Cochrane Database Syst Rev.* (3): CD005470.

CASP (2014) CASP checklists. CASP: Oxford. www.casp-uk.net/#!casp-tools-checklists/ c18f8 (accessed 22 June 2014).

Charlton BG, Miles A (1998) The rise and fall of EBM. *QJM.* **91**(5): 371–4.

Choudhry NK, Fletcher RH, Soumerai SB (2005) Systematic review: the relationship between clinical experience and quality of health care. *Ann Intern Med.* **142**(4): 260–73.

Cooksey D (2006) *A review of UK health research funding.* The Stationery Office: London.

Covell DG, Uman GC, Manning PR (1985) Information needs in office practice: are they being met? *Ann Intern Med.* **103**(4): 596–9.

Dickersin K (1990) The existence of publication bias and risk factors for its occurrence. *JAMA.* **263**(10): 1385–9.

Easterbrook PJ, Berlin JA, Gopalan R, *et al.* (1991) Publication bias in clinical research. *Lancet.* **337**(8746): 867–72.

Ernst E (2002) A systematic review of systematic reviews of homeopathy. *Br J Clin Pharmacol.* **54**(6): 577–82.

Gill P, Dowell AC, Neal RD, *et al.* (1996) Evidence based general practice: a retrospective study of interventions in one training practice. *BMJ.* **312**(7034): 819–21.

Gillam S, Siriwardena AN (2010) *The Quality and Outcomes Framework: QOF transforming general practice.* Radcliffe Publishing: Oxford.

Gillam SJ, Siriwardena AN, Steel N (2012) Pay-for-performance in the United Kingdom: impact of the quality and outcomes framework – a systematic review. *Ann Fam Med.* **10**(5): 461–8.

Greenhalgh T, Howick J, Maskrey N (2014) Evidence based medicine a movement in crisis? *BMJ.* **348**: g3725.

Korenstein D, McGinn T (2008) The impact of an intensive smoking cessation intervention. *Mt Sinai J Med.* **75**(6): 552–5.

NHS Centre for Reviews and Dissemination (1999) *Getting evidence into practice.* University of York: York.

Oxman AD, Thomson MA, Davis DA, *et al.* (1995) No magic bullets: a systematic review of 102 trials of interventions to improve professional practice. *CMAJ.* **153**(10): 1423–31.

Popay J, Williams G (1998) Qualitative research and evidence-based healthcare. *J R Soc Med.* **91**(Suppl. 35): 32–7.

Pope C, Mays N (2006) *Qualitative research in health care.* Blackwell / BMJ Books: Malden, MA.

Ramsey PG, Carline JD, Inui TS, *et al.* (1991) Changes over time in the knowledge base of practicing internists. *JAMA.* **266**(8): 1103–7.

Sackett DL (2000) *Evidence-based medicine: how to practice and teach EBM.* Churchill Livingstone: London.

Sackett DL, Rosenberg WM, Gray JA, *et al.* (2007) Evidence based medicine: what it is and what it isn't. 1996. *Clin Orthop Relat Res.* **455**: 3–5.

Scottish Intercollegiate Guidelines Network (2014) *SIGN 50: a guideline developer's handbook, Annex B.* SIGN: Edinburgh.

Siriwardena AN (2005) A voice for quality. *Qual Prim Care.* **13**: 179–81.

Straus SE, McAlister FA (2000) Evidence-based medicine: a commentary on common criticisms. *CMAJ.* **163**(7): 837–41.

CHAPTER 12

Individual practice and how to improve it

SUMMARY

- Individual practice needs to be developed to improve effectiveness, safety and patient experience.
- Although good systems can support better individual performance, without personal development individual practice can be a source of error.
- Models of competence and practice help us to understand the causes of good or poor practice.
- Quality improvement techniques can be used to improve individual practice and this can be incorporated into the appraisal process for doctors, nurses and other healthcare professionals.

INTRODUCTION

For many healthcare practitioners the main focus of their work is their individual practice involving face-to-face contact with patients. They are primarily concerned with how to improve the care they provide at a personal level.

In previous chapters we have considered how quality improvement efforts at a wider macro- (multi-organisational), meso- (organisational) and clinical micro-system affect individual practice, but in this chapter we focus on how practitioners can personally improve the care that they provide.

Although systems can be designed to improve quality and safety, a disproportionately large number of errors and failures have been shown to be attributable to a small minority of healthcare workers, an example of the Pareto principle, which suggests that 80% of errors come from 20% of practitioners (Bismark, *et al.* 2013).

FROM KNOWLEDGE TO PRACTICE

Improvement at an individual level is essentially based on learning, but this is not simply about acquiring knowledge. It also implies an ability to demonstrate the knowledge through the skill of applying this knowledge in practice and then the attitudes that lead to these skills being used consistently in day-to-day practice. This progression, from knowledge to its application and from demonstration of competence to performance, is captured in Miller's pyramid (*see* Figure 12.1) (Miller 1990)

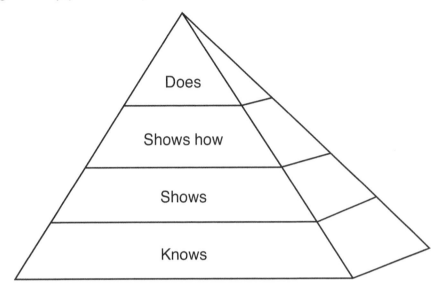

FIGURE 12.1 Miller's pyramid

THE SCOPE OF INDIVIDUAL PRACTICE

The scope and nature of clinical practice is neatly summarised by Norfolk's 'RDM-p' model, which incorporates relationship, diagnostics, management and professionalism (*see* Figure 12.2) (Norfolk and Siriwardena 2009).

Relationships with patients, relatives and carers, professionals and even members of the public are central to clinical work and depend on good communication skills, and other attributes such as empathy, which leads to trust.

'Diagnostics' refers to gathering, interpreting and prioritising information to decision-making, which includes the clinical diagnostic process, but also more widely to decisions we make in day-to-day practice. The cognitive processes at each stage of the 'diagnostic journey' determine the accuracy and safety of our decision-making.

Management is primarily about how effectively we tackle work processes and tasks, how efficiently and reliably we carry out our responsibilities – whether administrative activities such as dealing with prescriptions, tests results and correspondence, or conducting a consultation, or dealing with multiple (sometimes conflicting) priorities.

Management is also about monitoring ourselves effectively, maintaining both our performance and our health.

Finally, professionalism is the glue that binds relationship, diagnostics and management together. It defines our commitment to best practice, with an emphasis on showing respect for people, acting responsibly and demonstrating ethical and moral behaviour.

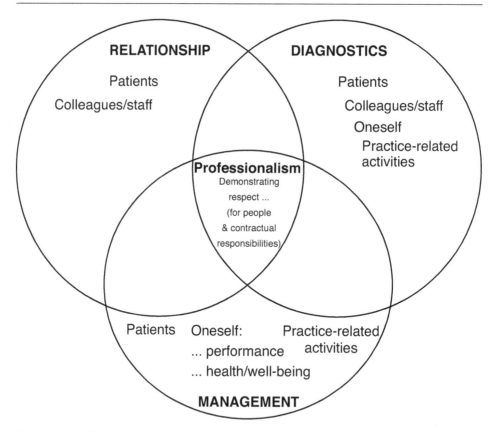

FIGURE 12.2 Relationship, Diagnostics, Management and professionalism (RDM-p) (Norfolk and Siriwardena 2009) © Tim Norfolk

THE CAUSES OF POOR PRACTICE

The RDM-p model identifies the nature of clinical practice, and where strengths or potential difficulties may arise. The model is then revisited when considering the causes of good (or poor) practice, specifically to assess whether weaknesses in skills and/or knowledge have contributed to relationship, management or diagnostics problems, and similarly whether poor attitudes (i.e. professionalism) have influenced outcomes. This deeper analysis of causal factors is described in a separate model, developed by Norfolk through painstaking analysis of medical underperformance: the SKIPE model – skills, knowledge, internal, past and external factors (Norfolk and Siriwardena 2013).

In the SKIPE model (*see* Figure 12.3), skills and knowledge form the bedrock of competence, but their application can be affected by other internal factors such as attitudes, personality and health, or external factors such as the work or non-work environment.

Improvement implies that we assess our strengths and weaknesses in a systematic way. These models enable us to consider our strengths and weaknesses more broadly and thus to build on our strengths and address our weaknesses.

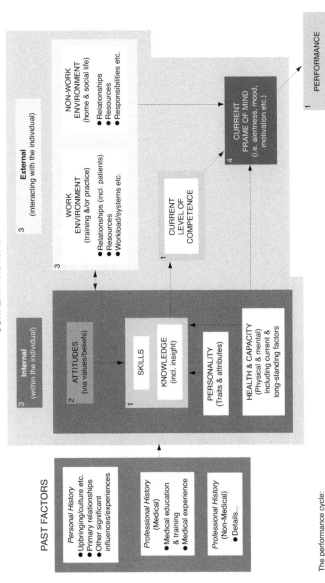

CURRENT FACTORS

PAST FACTORS

Personal History
●Upbringing/culture etc.
●Primary relationships
●Other significant
influences/experiences

Professional History
(Medical)
●Medical education
& training
●Medical experience

Professional History
(Non-Medical)
●Details...

3 **Internal**
(within the individual)

2 ATTITUDES
(via values/beliefs)

1 SKILLS

KNOWLEDGE
(incl. insight)

PERSONALITY
(Traits & attributes)

HEALTH & CAPACITY
(Physical & mental)
Including current &
long-standing factors

3 **External**
(interacting with the individual)

3 WORK
ENVIRONMENT
(training &/or practice)
●Relationships (incl. patients)
●Resources
●Workload/systems etc.

NON-WORK
ENVIRONMENT
(home & social life)
●Relationships
●Resources
●Responsibilities etc.

1 CURRENT
LEVEL OF
COMPETENCE

4 CURRENT
FRAME OF MIND
(i.e. alertness, mood,
motivation etc.)

1 PERFORMANCE

© Tim Norfolk

The performance cycle:

1. 'Primary' cycle: (a) skills & knowledge define competence, which determines performance; (b) flaws in performance addressed by
strengthening knowledge & skills, which (c) redefines competence...etc.
2. Respect/importance attached to tasks/responsibilities determines priority given to developing and demonstrating knowledge & skills
3. Current internal & external factors potentially influence development & demonstration of knowledge & skills
4. Individual's 'mindset' at any given moment, essentially determined by Internal & External factors, 'mediates' relationship between
current competence and performance

FIGURE 12.3 SKIPE model of causal factors potentially influencing medical performance (Norfolk and Siriwardena 2013) © Tim Norfolk

APPRAISAL AND REVALIDATION

Currently, the main focus for health professionals thinking strategically about their own learning needs is through periodic, formalised appraisal. Appraisal is a process for constructive dialogue in which the health professional being appraised has a formal structured opportunity to reflect on his or her work and to consider how his or her effectiveness might be improved. It is an opportunity to give feedback on past performance, to chart continuing progress and to identify future development needs.

The primary aim of appraisal is to help health professionals consolidate and improve on good performance. In doing so, it helps to identify areas where further development may be necessary or useful. It can help to identify problems of performance at an early stage; and also to recognise factors that may have led to poor performance, such as ill health (*see* Box 12.1).

BOX 12.1 Aims of appraisal

- Set out personal and professional development needs and agree plans for these to be met
- Review regularly an individual's work and performance, using relevant and appropriate comparative operational data from local, regional and national sources
- Consider the individual's contribution to the quality and improvement of services delivered locally
- Optimise the use of skills and resources to achieve the delivery of general and personal medical services
- Identify the resources needed to meet service objectives in the agreed job plan
- Discuss and seek support for an individual's participation in activities for the wider National Health Service
- Utilise the annual appraisal process and associated documentation to meet professional registration requirements (e.g. for General Medical Council or Nursing and Midwifery Council revalidation)

Appraisal underpins continuing professional development and provides doctors and nurses with an opportunity to demonstrate the evidence required for future revalidation. While appraisal is formative, revalidation is a summative process.

Revalidation involves a judgement as to whether a doctor is fit to practise and should remain on the medical register. The revalidation process informs the General Medical Council's decision on whether to renew an individual's registration and this currently occurs every 5 years. The Nursing and Midwifery Council is currently consulting on the corresponding processes for nurses.

HOW APPRAISAL WORKS

Appraisal is personal; its purpose is to support individual development (Middlemass and Siriwardena 2003). The process should be developmental, rigorously conducted and well informed. That means adequate preparation time, both by appraiser and appraisee (Chambers, *et al.* 2003). Its prime focus is on how patient care can be improved.

The content of medical appraisal was originally based on the core domains set out in the General Medical Council's *Good Medical Practice* document, together with consideration of the doctor's contribution to meeting local patient needs (*see* Box 12.2).

BOX 12.2 General Medical Council core headings

Knowledge, skills and performance
- Develop and maintain your professional performance
- Apply knowledge and experience to practice
- Record your work clearly, accurately and legibly

Safety and quality
- Contribute to and comply with systems to protect patients
- Respond to risks to safety
- Protect patients and colleagues from any risk posed by your health

Communication, partnership and teamwork
- Communicate effectively
- Work collaboratively with colleagues to maintain or improve patient care
- Teaching, training, supporting and assessing
- Continuity and coordination of care
- Establish and maintain partnerships with patients

Maintaining trust
- Show respect for patients
- Treat patients and colleagues fairly and without discrimination
- Act with honesty and integrity

BEING APPRAISED: THE PROCESS

Appraisees need to consider their priorities, reflect on practice over the previous year, choose appropriate tools or portfolios to help this review, and prepare a submission for the appraiser. At interview, progress is charted beginning with a review of last year's personal development plan (PDP). Personal learning needs are identified and a learning plan is generated. The appraiser should provide feedback that is honest, sensitive and encouraging.

Prompts to reflection include reviews of significant event logs, audits, complaints, case reviews, prescribing or other activity data. More personalised insights into the way you practise can stem from multidisciplinary peer review (multisource or 360-degree feedback). Health professionals are strongly encouraged to measure their patients' satisfaction using validated questionnaires.

The key points of the discussion and outcome must be fully documented. Appraiser and appraisee must complete and sign the appraisal summary statement and send a copy, in confidence, to the relevant responsible officer. Electronic portfolios greatly facilitate this process. All records must be held on a secure basis compliant with the requirements of the Data Protection Act 1998.

If it becomes apparent, during the appraisal process, that there is a potentially serious performance issue that requires further action, the appraiser must refer the matter immediately to the senior appraiser or responsible officer. This may culminate in referral to other sources of support.

IMPROVING INDIVIDUAL PERFORMANCE

In previous chapters we have described how performance can be improved at organisational or multi-organisational levels using quality improvement and change management techniques and skills. Quality improvement projects can also be effectively used to improve individual performance and can be used as part of the appraisal process (*see* Box 12.3) (Siriwardena 2011).

BOX 12.3 Quality improvement projects

Description of a quality improvement programme should include the:
- title of the quality improvement programme
- reason for the choice of topic and statement of the problem
- process under consideration (process mapping)
- priorities for improvement and the measurements adopted
- techniques used to improve the processes
- baseline data collection, analysis and presentation
- quality improvement objectives
- intervention and the maintenance of successful changes
- quality improvement achieved and reflections on the process in terms of:
  - knowledge, skills and performance
  - safety and quality
  - communication, partnership and teamwork
  - maintaining trust.

BOX 12.4 Example of an individual quality improvement project

Title: Improving individual referral letter accuracy, timeliness and completion

Date completed: 1 May 2010

Description: A quality improvement project focusing on improving the accuracy, timeliness and completion of specialist referral letters.

Reason for the choice of topic and statement of the problem: The project was triggered by a significant event involving a delayed referral letter for a patient. Fortunately, the patient did not come to any harm but it became apparent to me that my processes for completing referral letters needed to be safe, effective and efficient and there was no room for error or delay.

Process under consideration (process mapping): Current processes for referral letters were reviewed. This involved producing a list of referrals when they were indicated; dictating the letter on a tape after each surgery or dictating the letter directly to a secretary if the doctor was available and particularly for urgent letters; leaving the tape for the secretary to type and initiating an electronic booking with the specialist unit; and then signing the letter when next in the surgery or sometimes on the same day if an urgent referral was required. There were delays and potential for waste or error in this process, many of which had previously been experienced. For example, dictation machines and tapes or secretaries were not always available, batteries were sometimes missing from machines and tapes were sometimes damaged. Secretaries were not always able to understand what he had said on a tape, either, because it was damaged or because technical language was used that they did not understand. If a secretary was on leave or unwell there was a delay in the letter being typed. Inaccuracies in letters had to be corrected, necessitating retyping and leading to further delays.

Priorities for improvement and the measurements adopted: The aim of this quality improvement project was to improve the timeliness, accuracy and completion of referral letters. The steps required in the process and the potential for waste or error in the process were measured.

Baseline data collection, analysis and presentation: The baseline analysis was the process map of the steps involved in producing a referral letter and any risks or threats to a letter being sent described earlier.

Quality improvement objectives: The objective was to reduce the steps required to generate a referral letter and to minimise the potential for waste or error in the process.

Techniques used to improve the process: A process map and two plan-do-study-act (PDSA) cycles were used to improve the process of generating and sending referral letters. This was discussed with the secretaries and administrators. In the first PDSA, referral letters were typed directly onto the computer system after a surgery and the typed letter sent to the secretary as a computerised task (similar to an internal email on the clinical computer system). Letters were retyped on headed notepaper and a referral booking actioned by the secretary. In the second PDSA, letters were typed while the patient was in the room or just after he or she had left. This reduced the number of steps further and meant there was less to remember when generating a letter – sometimes the patient could be asked for salient information to include, prompted by the process of writing the letter.

Intervention and the maintenance of successful changes: The new process of typing referral letters with the patient present or just after he or she had left the room and sending them directly to the secretary as a computer task was implemented. This system has been maintained with benefits for the patient primarily but also for the doctor, secretaries and administrative staff.

Quality improvement achieved and reflections on the process in terms of knowledge, skills and performance; safety and quality; communication, partnership and teamwork; maintaining trust: This quality improvement project enabled the doctor to refine the process of generating referral letters. Letters are now generated with the patient present or just after the consultation. Patients are pleased that referral letters are sent immediately and when they have an opportunity to be involved in the content of the letter. Secretaries have fewer difficulties interpreting damaged tapes or difficult jargon and are more confident with the new process. The new process saves time, reduces errors and minimises waste or rework (having to do things twice or several times).

The models described here enable us to assess individual practice, to identify and address problems, and to improve individual practice through the use of quality improvement techniques, which can provide evidence for appraisal and revalidation.

CONCLUSION

In this chapter we have examined models for understanding the scope, nature and determinants of individual practice. We have also described how to apply improvement science to personal improvement.

Quality improvement and safety are now essential knowledge for healthcare staff in medicine, nursing and allied health professions. The processes of appraisal and revalidation will form a central part of their working lives.

REFERENCES

Bismark MM, Spittal MJ, Gurrin LC, *et al.* (2013) Identification of doctors at risk of recurrent complaints: a national study of healthcare complaints in Australia. *BMJ Qual Saf.* 22(7): 532–40.

Chambers R, Wakley G, Field S, *et al.* (2003) *Appraisal for the apprehensive: a guide for doctors.* Radcliffe Publishing: Oxford.

Middlemass J, Siriwardena AN (2003) General practitioners, revalidation and appraisal: a cross sectional survey of attitudes, beliefs and concerns in Lincolnshire. *Med Educ.* 37(9): 778–85.

Miller GE (1990) The assessment of clinical skills/competence/performance. *Acad Med.* 65(9 Suppl.): S63–7.

Norfolk T, Siriwardena AN (2013) A comprehensive model for diagnosing the causes of individual medical performance problems: skills, knowledge, internal, past and external factors (SKIPE). *Qual Prim Care.* 21(5): 315–23.

Norfolk T, Siriwardena AN (2009) A unifying theory of clinical practice: Relationship, Diagnostics, Management and professionalism (RDM-p). *Qual Prim Care.* 17(1): 37–47.

Siriwardena AN (2011) Quality improvement projects for appraisal and revalidation of general practitioners. *Qual Prim Care.* 19(4): 205–9.

Conclusion

In the preceding chapters we have attempted to provide readers with an introduction to the science of quality improvement (QI), implementation and
safety.

In the first section we examined the fundamental importance of patient perspectives on quality, together with contextual levers for improvement such as
leadership and management, regulation and commissioning.

In the second section we included chapters on QI tools and techniques, the
foundations of which are improvement frameworks and models, which led to
discussion of processes, their measurement and spreading improvement using
the features of healthcare systems.

In the third and final section we examined the evaluation of improvement
initiatives, evidence-based healthcare, the translation of evidence into practice
and how to apply improvement science to personal development.

One aim of this book has been to develop your understanding of QI.
However, you cannot develop skills purely by accumulating knowledge: you
need experience of the activities we have described. A useful next step is to consider the opportunities that your current role offers you to develop practical
competency in QI. These might include undertaking a specific audit or QI project, joining or heading a project team, or chairing a clinical governance group.

To learn as much as possible from this, you need to review your experience
systematically. Keep a personal learning diary, noting important lessons. Which
approaches worked best, in which situations? What were people's reactions to
your input? Seek feedback on your performance from your colleagues.

As we have seen, successful QI requires leadership and management. There
is no right or wrong way to manage. Management – like medicine – is not an
exact science. One high-profile medical manager defined a sense of humour,
intelligence and listening skills as the three most crucial attributes for a successful clinician manager (Chantler 1989). Adopting an appropriate management
'style' involves accurately analysing your organisation's circumstances, assessing
the needs of the people reporting to you and to whom you report, identifying
your own preferred approach, and adjusting this to the needs of the situation.

You can learn a lot from the behaviour of those who are acknowledged to
be effective leaders. Observe the leaders in your organisation. Do they convey a
sense of mission to their colleagues? If so, how? What differences in approach
can you detect between those who do and those who do not?

Most primary care professionals work in groups or teams. Membership of
a team can exert surprising influences over people's behaviour – both positive
and negative! As members of a group, people will reach decisions and take

actions that as individuals they would never dream of. If you regard people only as individuals, then as a manager you are ignoring some of the most significant and powerful influences that determine how well, or how badly, they will work.

Therefore, QI leaders must be acutely aware of the nature of groups, of the impact they can have on individuals, and of how to manage working groups so as to get the best out of them. Your task is to influence groups so that they apply their efforts to the attainment of organisational goals.

QI, safety and implementation science are rapidly becoming essential knowledge for healthcare staff in medicine, nursing and allied health professions. We hope this book has whetted your appetite to learn more.

REFERENCE

Chantler C (1989) Be a manager. *BMJ.* **298**(6686): 1505–8.

Additional online resources

Clinical Audit Support Centre (*see* 'What is Clinical Audit?'): www.clinical auditsupport.com/what_is_clinical_audit.html

Critical Appraisal Skills Programme: www.casp-uk.net

Doctors.net.uk: www.doctors.net.uk

Faculty of Medical Leadership and Management: www.fmlm.ac.uk

General Medical Council (*see* 'GMC Questionnaires and Resources'): www. gmc-uk.org/doctors/revalidation/colleague_patient_feedback_resources.asp

Health and Social Care Information Centre: www.hscic.gov.uk/

Healthcare Quality Improvement Partnership: www.hqip.org.uk/

The Health Foundation: www.health.org.uk

Institute for Healthcare Improvement: www.ihi.org

The King's Fund: www.kingsfund.org.uk

National Institute for Health and Care Excellence: www.nice.org.uk

NHS England – Patient Safety (*see* 'Healthcare Risk Assessment Made Easy'): www.nrls.npsa.nhs.uk/resources/?EntryId45=59825

NHS Evidence: www.evidence.nhs.uk

NHS Improving Quality – The Productive series: www.institute.nhs.uk/quality_ and_value/productivity_series/the_productive_series.html

Self Management UK: http://selfmanagementuk.org/

UK Cochrane Centre: http://ukcc.cochrane.org

Glossary

absolute risk The observed or calculated probability of an event in the population under study

absolute risk reduction The difference in the absolute risk (rates of adverse events) between study and control populations

action research Research that involves participants to a greater or lesser extent in the conception, design and evaluation of an intervention designed to bring about change

acute myocardial infarction (AMI) A condition causing symptoms including chest pain or sudden death due to complete blockage of a coronary artery

adjustment A summarising procedure for a statistical measure in which the effects of differences in composition of the populations being compared have been minimised by statistical methods

aetiology The study of the causes of disease

appraisal The (annual) formal structured process for a person to reflect on his or her work and to consider how his or her effectiveness might be improved

association Statistical dependence between two or more events, characteristics or other variables; an association may be fortuitous or may be produced by various other circumstances; the presence of an association does not necessarily imply a causal relationship

attributable risk The proportion of the risk of a disease that can be attributed to a named causal factor

audit (clinical) The systematic measurement of performance and implementation of change against one or more predefined criteria against a standard until that standard is achieved or until a new standard is set

bias (*synonym: systematic error*) Deviation of results or inferences from the truth, or processes leading to such deviation (*see* also 'selection bias')

binomial distribution The probability distribution of the number of successes in a sequence of n independent yes/no experiments, each of which yields success with probability p

blind(ed) study (*synonym: masked study*) A study in which observer(s) and/ or subjects are kept ignorant of the group to which the subjects are assigned, as in an experimental study, or of the population from which the subjects come, as in a non-experimental or observational study; where both observer and subjects are kept ignorant, the study is termed a double-blind study; if the statistical analysis is also done in ignorance of the group to which subjects belong, the study is sometimes described as triple blind; the purpose of 'blinding' is to eliminate sources of bias

Bristol Royal Infirmary scandal A public inquiry into children's heart surgery chaired by Sir Ian Kennedy into deaths of babies during cardiac surgery at Bristol Royal Infirmary between 1990 and 1995; the inquiry found staff shortages, a lack of leadership and that the unit was 'simply not up to the task'

Care Quality Commission (CQC)   The independent regulator responsible for the quality and safety regulator of all health and social care services in England

case–control study   Retrospective comparison of exposures of persons with disease (cases) with those of persons without the disease (controls) (*see* 'retrospective study')

case fatality rate   The proportion of people with a disease who die within a defined period from diagnosis

case series   Report of a number of cases of disease

case study   A research design based on a single case or multiple cases that combines qualitative and quantitative methods to provide a descriptive, exploratory or explanatory analysis of a person, group or event

causality   The relating of causes to the effects they produce; most of epidemiology concerns causality and several types of causes can be distinguished (it must be emphasised, however, that epidemiological evidence by itself is insufficient to establish causality, although it can provide powerful circumstantial evidence)

cause and effect ('fishbone' or Ishikawa) diagram   A diagram representing the patient pathway leading to the outcome of interest and how this is affected by various inputs, including people, providers, processes, equipment and policies

clinical audit   *See* 'audit (clinical)'

clinical commissioning groups (CCGs)   The primary care-led organisations set up by the Health and Social Care Act 2012 to organise the delivery of National Health Service services in England

clinical governance   The framework through which National Health Service organisations and their staff are accountable for the quality of patient care

clinical microsystem   A system comprising groups of clinicians interacting to provide specific types of care for patients

Cochrane Review   A systematic review of primary research in human healthcare and health policy, undertaken to the highest standard

cohort study   Follow-up of exposed and non-exposed defined groups, with a comparison of disease rates during the time covered

commissioning   The planning and purchasing of health services

common cause variation   Natural random predictable variation occurring over time in a process that is inherent to the elements contributing to that process

co-morbidity   Coexistence of a disease or diseases in a study participant in addition to the index condition that is the subject of study

comparison group   Any group to which the index group is compared; usually synonymous with control group

complex systems   Systems incorporating multiple components and multiple interactions that can lead to non-linear and unpredictable rather than simple linear cause and effect reactions to stimuli

confidence interval (CI)   The range of numerical values in which we can be confident (to a computed probability, such as 90% or 95%) that the population value being estimated will be found; confidence intervals indicate the strength of evidence; where confidence intervals are wide, they indicate less precise estimates of effect; the larger the trial's sample size, the larger the number of outcome events and the greater becomes the confidence that the true relative risk reduction is close to the value stated; this is not the same as a control limit

confounding variable, confounder   A variable that can cause or prevent the outcome of interest, is not an intermediate variable, and is associated with the factor under investigation; a confounding variable may be due to chance or bias; unless it is possible to adjust for confounding variables, their effects cannot be distinguished from those of factor(s) being studied

control chart   A graph that plots numbers or rates of a process over time showing the mean and control limits to determine the nature of variation in that process

control limits   The limits of common cause variation in a stable process calculated according to the data and its distribution

Creutzfeldt–Jakob disease   A rare, fatal condition affecting the brain caused by an abnormal infectious protein called a prion

criterion   A measurable aspect of quality (structure, process or outcome) of care

critical-to-quality tree   The measurable characteristics of a process, where standards need to be achieved to meet the quality requirements of the user

demography   The study of human populations

determinant   Any definable factor that effects a change in a health condition or other characteristic

disability   In the context of health experience a disability is any restriction or lack (resulting from an impairment) of ability to perform an activity in the manner or within the range considered normal for a human being

disability-adjusted life year   A method of calculating the health impact of a disease in terms of the cases of premature death, disability and days of infirmity due to illness from a specific disease or condition

dose–response relationship   A relationship in which change in amount, intensity or duration of exposure is associated with a change – either an increase or decrease – in risk of a specified outcome

driver diagram   A graphical depiction of a logical set of underpinning goals ('primary drivers') and specific actions ('secondary drivers') needed to bring about a high-level improvement goal

effectiveness   A measure of the benefit resulting from an intervention for a given health problem under usual conditions of clinical care for a particular group; this form of evaluation considers both the efficacy of an intervention and its acceptance by those to whom it is offered, answering the question, 'Does the practice do more good than harm to people to whom it is offered?' (*see* 'intention to treat' analysis)

efficacy   A measure of the benefit resulting from an intervention for a given health problem under the ideal conditions of an investigation; it answers the question, 'Does the practice do more good than harm to people who fully comply with the recommendations?'

environmental health   The theory and practice of assessing, correcting, controlling, and preventing those factors in the environment that can potentially affect adversely the health of present and future generations

epidemic   The occurrence of disease at higher than expected levels; this could be an endemic disease at higher than usual levels or non-endemic disease at any level

epidemiology   The study of the distribution and determinants of health-related states or events in specified populations, and the application of this study to control of health problems

evaluation   A process that attempts to determine as systematically and objectively as possible the relevance, effectiveness and impact of activities in the light of their objectives

evidence-based healthcare / medicine / public health   Systematic use of evidence derived from published research

exclusion criteria   Conditions that preclude entrance of candidates into an investigation even if they meet the inclusion criteria

follow-up   Observation over a period of time of an individual, group or initially defined population whose relevant characteristics have been assessed in order to observe changes in health status or health-related variables

forcefield analysis   An analysis of barriers and facilitators of change

funnel plot (trombonogram)   A graph that compares organisational units at a single point or during a fixed period of time by plotting the percentage success of a process across organisational units

General Medical Services contract   The detailed agreement between the UK government and general practitioners of the services they will provide under the National Health Service

gold standard   A method, procedure, or measurement that is widely accepted as being the best available

Hawthorne effect   A change in a process or measure that results from a change in behaviour due to being observed

health   The extent to which an individual or a group is able to realise aspirations and satisfy needs, and to change or cope with the environment; health is a resource for everyday life, not the objective of living; it is a positive concept, emphasising social and personal resources as well as physical capabilities; your health is related to how much you feel your potential, to be a meaningful part of the society in which you find yourself, is adequately realised

health equity audit   A technique to identify how fairly services or other resources are distributed in relation to the health needs of different population groups or geographical areas

health improvement   The theory and practice of promoting the health of populations by influencing lifestyle and socio-economic, physical and cultural environment through methods of health promotion, directed towards populations, communities and individuals

health inequality   Differences observed between groups due to one group experiencing an advantage over the other group rather than to any innate differences between them

health inequity   The presence of unfair and avoidable or remedial differences in health among populations or groups defined socially

health promotion   The process of enabling people to exert control over and to improve their health; as well as covering actions aimed at strengthening people's skills and capabilities, it also includes actions directed towards changing social, environmental conditions to prevent or to improve their impact on individual and public health

impairment   In the context of health experience, an impairment is any loss or abnormality of psychological, physiological or anatomical structure or function

improvement science   Improvement science, also quality improvement and translational research, is the scientific study of quality improvement, ensuring that quality improvement is itself based on the best available evidence

incidence   The rate at which new cases occur in a population: the number of new cases of illness commencing, or of persons falling ill, during a specified time period in a given population (*see* also 'prevalence')

infant mortality   The proportion of live births that die up to 1 year of age

infection (colonisation)   This occurs when an organism enters the body, multiplies; it may be termed infection when damage is caused and colonisation when no damage is caused to the host; acute infection implies a short-lived infection with short period of infectivity; chronic infection refers to a persistent condition with ongoing replication of the organism; latent infection refers to a persistent infection with intermittent replication of the organism

healthcare innovation   A set of planned and coordinated actions to implement novel behaviours, routines or ways of working seeking to improve health outcomes, administrative efficiency, cost-effectiveness or users' experiences

innovation diffusion   The mechanism and process of spread of an innovation

intention to treat analysis   A method for data analysis in a randomised clinical trial in which individual outcomes are analysed according to the group to which they have been randomised, even if they never received the treatment they were assigned; by simulating practical experience it provides a better measure of effectiveness (versus efficacy)

interviewer bias   Systematic error due to interviewer's subconscious or conscious gathering of selective data

lead-time bias   Lead-time bias occurs when detection by screening seems to increase disease free survival but this is only because disease has been detected earlier and not because screening is delaying death or disease; if in a prognosis study patients are not all enrolled at similar, well-defined points in the course of their disease, differences in outcome over time may merely reflect differences in duration of illness

lean manufacturing   Lean manufacturing, enterprise or production, sometimes simply called 'lean', entails assessing every process for its value to the consumer, eliminating waste and improving efficiency

length-time bias   Length-time bias occurs if a screening programme is better at picking up milder forms of the disease; this means that people who develop disease that progresses more quickly or is more likely to be fatal are less likely to be picked up by screening and their outcomes may not be included in evaluations of the programme – thus the programme looks to be more effective than it is

life expectancy   The average number of additional years a person could expect to live if current mortality trends were to continue for the rest of that person's life; general given as a life expectancy from birth

lifelong learning   The process of continuing professional development or learning

likelihood ratio   Ratio of the probability that a given diagnostic test result will be expected for a patient with the target disorder rather than for a patient without the disorder

logic model   A logic model is a graphical representation of the causal relationships between the problem, population and priorities for change, the inputs (resources and activities) designed to bring about change and the resulting outputs and outcomes of a programme being designed or evaluated

maternal mortality ratio   The number of deaths during pregnancy and up to 42 days after delivery, per 100 000 live births

Mid Staffordshire NHS Foundation Trust public inquiry   The public inquiry chaired by Robert Francis QC into the role of the commissioning, supervisory and regulatory bodies in the monitoring of the Mid Staffordshire Foundation NHS Trust after the serious failings found in care of patients at the hospital; the public inquiry is established under the Inquiries Act 2005

Miller's pyramid   A diagram showing the progression from knowledge ('knowing') to its application ('knowing how') and from demonstration of competence ('showing how') to performance ('doing')

mixed methods research   An approach that combines and integrates multiple rigorous quantitative and qualitative methods to answer research questions that call for real-life contextual understandings of a phenomenon

model for improvement   The model considers what we are trying to achieve, how we will know if we have improved and what changes we can make to improve

Monitor   Monitor is the sector regulator for health services in England that has a role to protect and promote the interests of patients

morbidity   The impact of a disease that is not death; measures of morbidity include incidence and prevalence rates

mortality (rate)   Death; the number of deaths in an area as a proportion of the number of people in that area

National Health Service (NHS)   The UK National Health Service, which was established in 1948 to provide healthcare to the population free at the point of delivery

National Institute for Health and Care Excellence (NICE)   NICE provides independent, authoritative and evidence-based guidance for the National Health Service, local authorities, charities and all those responsible for commissioning or providing healthcare, public health or social care services to ensure that care is of the best possible quality and offers the best value for money

natural networks   A web of individuals or organisations together with the social interactions between them

need   These may be expressed by action (e.g. visiting a doctor) or felt needs (e.g. what people consider and/or say they need); the need for healthcare is often defined as the capacity to benefit from that care

negative predictive value (of a diagnostic or screening test)   The proportion of persons who test negative for a disease who, as measured by the gold standard, are identified as non-diseased

neonatal mortality   The proportion of live births who die within the first 28 days

normal (Gaussian) distribution   A continuous probability distribution that describes the probability that any real observation will fall between any two real limits as the curve approaches zero on either side

number needed to harm   The number of patients who must be exposed to an intervention before one unintended adverse outcome of the intervention occurs

number needed to treat   The number of patients who must be exposed to an intervention before the clinical outcome of interest occurred; for example, the number of patients needed to treat to prevent one adverse outcome

odds   A proportion in which the numerator contains the number of times an event occurs and the denominator includes the number of times the event does not occur

odds ratio   A measure of the degree of association; for example, the odds of exposure among the cases compared with the odds of exposure among the controls

organisational culture   The set of norms, beliefs, principles and ways of behaving that together give an organisation its distinctive character

p-value   The probability (ranging from zero to one) that the null hypothesis is true which indicates whether the results observed in a study (or results more extreme) could have occurred by chance

pandemic   A global epidemic; this is sometimes used for a very large-scale epidemic

patient participation group   Patient participation groups include groups of volunteer patients with members of practice staff who meet regularly to discuss services and how they can be improved

PESTLE analysis   An analysis of political, environmental, social, technological, legal and environmental factors for change

plan-do-study-act (PDSA) cycle   A method involving repeated rapid, small-scale tests of change in an organisation involving deciding what to change and how to change it (plan), introducing the change (do), measuring its effects (study) and then after modifying the change (act), repeating the cycle of change

policy   An overall statement of the aims of an organisation within a particular context

Poisson distribution   The distribution describing the probability of a given number of events occurring in a fixed interval of time, space, distance, area or volume if these events occur with a known average rate and are independent of previous last event

population strategy   Targets preventive interventions at the whole population

positive predictive value (of a diagnostic or screening test)   The proportion of persons who test positive for a disease who, as measured by the gold standard, are identified as diseased

precision   The range in which the best estimates of a true value approximate the true value (*see* 'confidence interval')

predictive value   In screening and diagnostic tests, the probability that a person with a positive test is a true positive (i.e. does have the disease), or that a person with a negative test truly does not have the disease; the predictive value of a screening test is determined by the sensitivity and specificity of the test, and by the prevalence of the condition for which the test is used

prevalence   The proportion of persons with a particular disease within a given population at a given time; point prevalence is the prevalence at one single point in time; period prevalence is the proportion of persons with a particular disease over a specified period of time

prevention   Primary prevention: actions designed to prevent the occurrence of the problem (e.g. health education, immunisation)

Secondary prevention: actions designed to detect and treat the occurrence of a problem before symptoms have developed (e.g. screening, early diagnosis)

Tertiary prevention: actions designed to limit disability once a condition is manifest (e.g. limitation of disability, rehabilitation)

prevention paradox   Preventive measures bringing large benefits to the community offer little to each participating individual

primary care trust   Local National Health Service health authorities in England charged with improving health and commissioning healthcare

primary healthcare   First-contact care provided by a range of healthcare professionals, nurses, dentists, pharmacists, optometrists, and complementary therapists

process map   A tool to show pictorially the series of steps in a process of care or a patient journey

prognosis   The possible outcomes of a disease or condition and the likelihood that each one will occur

prognostic factor   Demographic, disease-specific or co-morbid characteristics associated strongly enough with a condition's outcomes to predict accurately the eventual development of those outcomes; compare with risk factors; neither prognostic nor risk factors necessarily imply a cause and effect relationship

prospective study   Study design where one or more groups (cohorts) of individuals who have not yet had the outcome event in question are monitored for the number of such events that occur over time

public health   The science and art of preventing disease, prolonging life, and promoting health through the organised efforts and informed choices of society, organisations, public and private, communities and individuals; public health practice is the emphasis in this book, while public health may also be considered as a discipline or a social institution

qualitative   Research methods including interviews, focus groups and other designs that aim to elicit an in-depth understanding of human behaviour and to generate hypotheses about how and why behaviour occurs

quality-adjusted life year   A health measure that combines the quantity and quality of life; it takes 1 year of perfect health-life expectancy to be worth 1 and regards 1 year of less than perfect life expectancy as less than 1

Quality and Outcomes Framework (QOF)   The national primary care pay-for-performance (P4P) scheme in the United Kingdom

quality improvement collaborative (QIC)   Multi-organisational, multi-professional initiatives in which improvement and clinical experts, using structured activities, engage clinicians to effect improvement in a specific area of practice

quantitative   Research methods including cross-sectional surveys, case–control, cohort and experimental designs which usually aim to test hypotheses

randomised controlled trial (RCT)   Study design where treatments, interventions, or enrolment into different study groups are assigned by random allocation rather than by conscious decisions of clinicians or patients; if the sample size is large enough, this study design avoids problems of bias and confounding variables by assuring that both known and unknown determinants of outcome are evenly distributed between treatment and control groups

RDM-p model   A model of clinical practice which incorporates relationship, diagnostics, management and professionalism

recall bias   Systematic error due to the differences in accuracy or completeness of recall to memory of past events or experiences

relative risk (RR)   The ratio of the probability of developing, in a specified period of time, an outcome among those receiving the treatment of interest or exposed to a risk factor, compared with the probability of developing the outcome if the risk factor or intervention is not present

reliability (reproducibility repeatability)   The results of a test, measure or intervention are identical or closely similar each time it is conducted

retrospective study   Study design in which cases where individuals who had an outcome event in question are collected and analysed after the outcomes have occurred (*see* also 'case–control study')

revalidation   The process by which all licensed doctors are required to demonstrate once every 5 years that they are up to date and fit to practise

risk   The number of cases of a disease that occur in a defined period of time as a proportion of the number of people in the population at the beginning of the period

risk communication   The open two-way exchange of information and opinion about risk, leading to better understanding and better decisions about clinical management

risk factor   Patient characteristics or factors associated with an increased probability of developing a condition or disease in the first place; compare with prognostic factors; neither risk nor prognostic factors necessarily imply a cause and effect relationship

root cause analysis (RCA)   A method to identify the underlying causes of problems

run chart   A graph that plots dots of numbers or rates of a process over time with a median value to determine the nature of variation in that process

screening   A public health service in which members of a defined population, who do not necessarily perceive they are at risk of, or are already affected by, a disease or its complications, are asked a question or offered a test, to identify those individuals who are more likely to be helped than harmed by further tests or treatment to reduce the risk of a disease or its complications

secular trend   A trend over time, also termed temporal trend

selection bias   A bias in assignment or a confounding variable that arises from study design rather than by chance; these can occur when the study and control groups are chosen so that they differ from each other by one or more factors that may affect the outcome of the study.

  In screening selection bias occurs when the screening programme attracts people who are more or less likely to have the condition being screened for than the general population

sensitivity (of a diagnostic or screening test)   The proportion of truly diseased persons, as measured by the gold standard, who are identified as diseased by the test under study

Shipman inquiry   English GP Harold Shipman was convicted of murdering 15 of his patients in 2000 and is thought to have killed up to 250 of his patients; this led to the Shipman inquiry by Dame Janet Smith into the deaths

significant event analysis (SEA)   A method of audit that involves systematic and detailed review of 'significant' (either positive or negative) incidents identified by one or more members of the practice team, reflecting systematically on what occurred with the team and making recommendations for improvement

Six Sigma   Six Sigma refers to the limits for acceptable quality being set to include all observations within six standard deviations (sigma) of the mean in a normal distribution

SKIPE model   A model describing the causes of good or poor performance incorporating skills, knowledge, internal, past or external factors

social capital   Networks together with shared norms, values and understandings that facilitate cooperation within or among groups and which may thereby improve health

special cause variation   Non-random, unpredictable variation occurring over time in a process that is due to an assignable cause affecting that process (in contrast to common-cause variation)

specificity (of a diagnostic or screening test)   The proportion of truly non-diseased persons, as measured by the gold standard, who are identified as non-diseased by the test under study

standard   The threshold of expected compliance for a criterion usually expressed as a percentage

statistical process control   A statistical method used to analyse variation over time or between organisational units of any process

strategy   A plan of action designed to achieve a series of objectives

stratification   Division into groups; stratification may also refer to a process to control for differences in confounding variables, by making separate estimates for groups of individuals who have the same values for the confounding variable

strength of inference   The likelihood that an observed difference between groups within a study represents a real difference rather than mere chance or the influence of confounding factors, based on both p-values and confidence intervals; strength of inference is weakened by various forms of bias and by small sample sizes

surveillance   The ongoing, systematic collection, collation and analysis of data and the prompt dissemination of the resulting information to those who need to know so that an action can result

survival curve   A graph of the number of events occurring over time or the chance of being free of these events over time; the events must be discrete and the time at which they occur must be precisely known; in most clinical situations, the chance of an outcome changes with time; in most survival curves the earlier follow-up periods usually include results from more patients than the later periods and are therefore more precise

Swiss cheese model   A model that shows how major errors can arise from multiple small defects (the 'holes')

system   A set of interdependent and interacting elements, whether people, organisations or processes that, together with the context in which they operate, seek to achieve a common aim

total quality management   Total quality management is an organisational approach to continuously improve the quality of products or services to customers

translational research   Research that seeks to implement the findings of basic research into clinical practice or organisational systems

transtheoretical model   The process of behaviour change in terms of different motivational states during adoption of an innovation from precontemplation (not yet ready for change) through contemplation (thinking about change), preparation (for change), action (to implement change) and finally maintenance of change

trigger tool   Tools that use a structured record review to measure the rate of harm or changes in harm in a variety of healthcare settings

validity   The extent to which a variable or intervention measures what it is supposed to measure or accomplishes what it is supposed to accomplish; the internal validity of a study refers to the integrity of the experimental design; the external validity (generalisability) of a study refers to the appropriateness by which its results can be applied to non-study patients or populations

years of life lost   Years of potential life relate to the average age at which deaths occur and the expected life span of the population so a measure of how many potential years are lost due to early death provides a measure of the relative importance of conditions in causing mortality

Index

Entries in *italics* denote figures; entries in **bold** denote tables and boxes.

CPD with Radcliffe

You can now use a selection of our books to achieve CPD (Continuing Professional Development) points through directed reading.

We provide a free online form and downloadable certificate for your appraisal portfolio. Look for the CPD logo and register with us at: www.radcliffehealth.com/cpd

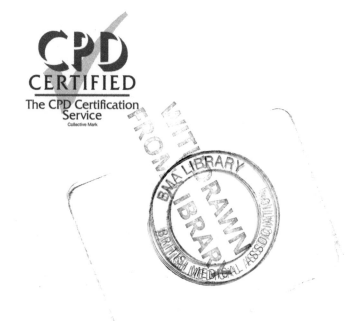